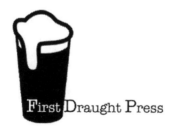

First Draught Press

Praise for *The Ventilator Book* from Amazon readers:

"It is a kitschy, fun read (never thought this was possible for something as dry as changing vent settings) - would be a great start for an intern, probably more that you would need to know. Reviews setting changes in a fun, memorable way."
　　—WonkaTron

"This is one of the best books I have ever read on ventilators. It's like a running commentary. It's concise, clear and full of realistic examples introduced at the right time (just before the concepts make you to start scratching your head). Of course as Dr. Owens admits, there are many more detailed books on mechanical ventilation which you can read for more knowledge. This book is so "down to earth" that any beginner can make sense out of it and any expert would agree with what I just wrote above."
　　—Avatar

"Every resident should make their lives easier and get a copy of this book. I'm an RT and this makes perfect sense. It's simple if you actually know what you're doing...which this book explains how to do perfectly."
　　—Sara Elane

"Excellent review of the fundamentals. Great for ICU fellows up at night. An excellent review also for older attendings 25 years out from their fellowship (yours truly). Good illustrations of ventilator mode variables and excellent text giving sound reasoning for making choices and adjustments in common disease states."
　　—xhighbar

"As a surgical resident working in the ICU, this book was an excellent introduction into ventilator management. Its main strength is in the way it is written. It does not read like a typical textbook but in more of a personal tone. I've recommended it to all of my junior residents and I would recommend it to anyone who is looking to improve their understanding of ventilator management."
　　—SPM88

"Vents finally make sense! Recommend to all medical professionals with any confusion about vents, settings, etc."
　　—D

The Advanced Ventilator Book

William Owens, MD

First Draught Press
MMXVII

This book is dedicated to the fellows, residents, medical students, nurses, and respiratory therapists whom I have had the privilege to teach over the years. Medicine is neither art nor science, but rather a craft. It requires a commitment to excellence from a craftsman. Paying it forward is part of the deal. This work is my attempt to share what I've learned about critical care medicine with the next generation.

Writing a book is not an easy task, and neither is being a physician. I could not do it without the love and support of Lorien, my wife and fellow adventurer.

Table of Contents

Introduction

The Ventilator Book was written as a guide for students, residents, nurses, and respiratory therapists. It was written with the goal of being a quick reference and an easy-to-read overview of mechanical ventilation. Based on feedback from readers, I believe that it has accomplished its purpose.

The Advanced Ventilator Book aims to take the reader to the next level, while preserving the same format and structure that makes *The Ventilator Book* a useful reference. This is a book designed for clinicians with some experience in caring for critically ill patients who would like some guidance on how to manage cases of severe respiratory failure. I have written it with the assumption that the reader understands the basics of mechanical ventilation and the pathophysiology of critical illness or injury. The first two chapters get back to the basics, with an overview of oxygen delivery and the concept of permissive hypercapnia. Following this are chapters covering the titration of positive end-expiratory pressure; the management of the patient with severe bronchospasm; the use of prone positioning and therapeutic neuromuscular blockade; inhaled nitric oxide and prostacyclin; veno-venous extracorporeal life support; and a chapter on incorporating all of this into a treatment strategy.

One feature of *The Ventilator Book* was the emphasis on practical use. Many textbooks and articles describe the rationale for a particular mode of ventilation or therapy, but relatively few actually tell the reader how to do it. *The Advanced Ventilator Book* provides the same step-by-step guidance to help clinicians put these principles into practice.

The Advanced Ventilator Book also continues the original book's emphasis on support and lung protection rather than cure. No magic bullets are promised, as none exist. Mechanical ventilation for patients with severe respiratory failure has great potential to harm, and so the avoidance of preventable injury is stressed with each topic in the book. The bulk of critical care medicine is supportive in nature, and the treatment of acute respiratory failure is no exception.

Chapter 1

Oxygen Delivery and Consumption

Many textbooks on respiratory and critical care medicine begin with statements like, "Oxygen is the most necessary and basic building block of life." In clinical training, the early application of high-flow oxygen is taught as a life-saving maneuver in emergencies. In the emergency department and intensive care unit, much importance is placed on keeping the pulse oximeter reading over 90% (and usually over 95%); likewise, there is a compulsion to keep the PaO_2 in the normal range of 90-100 mm Hg.

At first glance, there is nothing wrong with this approach. Oxygen is indeed necessary for life, and avoiding hypoxemia is a core part of resuscitation. When treating patients with severe respiratory failure, however, attaining a normal PaO_2 may be either impossible or only possible by the application of injurious airway pressures. Therefore, a more complete understanding of oxygen delivery and consumption is necessary.

Oxygen Content

Each gram of hemoglobin can bind 1.34 mL of oxygen when fully saturated. A small amount of oxygen is also carried in

3

the plasma in its dissolved form. This is represented by the PaO_2. The solubility coefficient for oxygen in plasma is 0.003. Putting all of this together yields the oxygen content equation:

$$CaO_2 = 1.34 \times Hgb \times SaO_2 + [PaO_2 \times 0.003]$$

With normal hemoglobin of 15 g/dL, SaO_2 of 100%, and a PaO_2 of 100 mm Hg, the oxygen content of arterial blood is 20.4 mL O_2/dL blood. It is important to note that the contribution made by the dissolved oxygen ($PaO_2 \times 0.003$) is very small—0.3 mL O_2/dL blood. The hemoglobin binds 98.5% of the oxygen content. The fraction contributed by the dissolved oxygen is negligible. If the FiO_2 on the ventilator were increased to bring the PaO_2 up to 500 mm Hg (keeping the SaO_2 at 100%), only 1.2 mL O_2/dL blood would be added to the oxygen content.

Keeping the PaO_2 elevated beyond what's necessary for adequate saturation of the hemoglobin is unlikely to be consequential except in cases of profound anemia (Hgb < 5 g/dL) or hyperbaric conditions. In fact, the PaO_2 can often be ignored when calculating oxygen content and delivery in order to make the math easier. This leads us to the first rule of oxygen: *The SaO_2 is what matters, not the PaO_2.*

Oxygen Delivery

Once the arterial blood is loaded with oxygen, it is delivered to the tissues to be used for metabolism. The amount of blood circulated per minute is the cardiac output, which is expressed in liters blood per minute. Since the CaO_2 is measured in deciliters, the units are converted by multiplying by 10. This yields the oxygen delivery equation:

$$DO_2 = CO \times CaO_2 \times 10$$

If a normal cardiac output is 5 L/min, the DO_2 is 1020 mL O_2/minute. In order to make comparisons among different patients of various heights and weights, this can be indexed by dividing the DO_2 by the body surface area. A "typical" body surface area is 1.7 m², so the "typical" DO_2I would be 1020/1.7, or 600 mL O_2/min/m².

The cardiac output has the greatest influence on oxygen delivery. Even during periods of arterial hypoxemia, an increase in cardiac output can be sufficient to deliver the necessary amount of oxygen to the tissues. The table below shows the effect that an increase in cardiac output can have on oxygen delivery, even with significant anemia or hypoxemia. It also shows that anemia has a more pronounced effect on oxygen delivery than hypoxemia. For the purposes of simplifying the calculations, the PaO_2 has been omitted. This leads us to the second rule of oxygen: *An increase in cardiac output can offset hypoxemia.*

Changes In Oxygen Delivery

CO	Hgb	SaO$_2$	DO$_2$
3 L/min	15 g/dL	100%	603 mL O$_2$/min
8 L/min	7 g/dL	100%	750 mL O$_2$/min
5 L/min	15 g/dL	100%	1005 mL O$_2$/min
8 L/min	15 g/dL	75%	1206 mL O$_2$/min

Oxygen Consumption

During periods of rest, the body's consumption of oxygen (VO_2) is approximately 200-250 mL O_2/minute. Indexed for body surface area, the resting VO_2I is 120-150 mL O_2/min/m². Normal subjects can increase their VO_2 during peak exercise by a factor of 10, and elite athletes can reach a maximum VO_2 of 20-25 times their resting consumption. During critical illnesses like septic shock, multisystem trauma, or burn injury, VO_2 increases over baseline by approximately 30-50%.

The consumption of oxygen by the tissues (VO_2) varies by organ system. The brain and heart consume the most delivered oxygen, while hair, bones, and nails consume a negligible amount. This can be further complicated by the fact that different organ systems receive different amounts of the cardiac output—the brain consumes the most oxygen, for example, but also receives 15% of the total blood flow. The coronary circulation, on the other hand, accounts for only 5% of the total cardiac output so the percentage of delivered oxygen that is consumed is much higher. Fortunately for the clinician, this is not important because regional monitoring of oxygen delivery and consumption is practical only in laboratory animals. Measurement of the total body VO_2, on the other hand, can be done rather easily with a pulmonary artery catheter (more accurate) or by using a combination of a noninvasive cardiac output monitor along with a measurement of central venous oxygen saturation (less accurate). While this is not as precise as directly measuring the content of oxygen in expired gas, it is a close enough approximation for clinical use.

By measuring the mixed venous oxygen saturation in the pulmonary artery, the venous oxygen content can be calculated:

$$CvO_2 = 1.34 \text{ x Hgb x } SvO_2 + [PvO_2 \text{ x } 0.003]$$

As with the arterial oxygen content equation, the minor contribution made by the dissolved oxygen (in this case, the PvO_2), can be omitted from the calculation. Thus, for a hemoglobin of 15 g/dL and a normal SvO_2 of 75%, the venous oxygen content is 15.1 mL O_2/dL blood. The difference between arterial and venous oxygen content is normally 3-5 mL O_2/dL blood.

The VO_2 can then be calculated by multiplying the arterial-venous oxygen difference by the cardiac output and converting units:

$$VO_2 = CO \times [CaO_2 - CvO_2] \times 10$$

Expanded, this equation is:

$$VO_2 = CO \times [(1.34 \times Hgb \times SaO_2)-(1.34 \times Hgb \times SvO_2)] \times 10$$

Rearranged (and simpler):

$$VO_2 = CO \times 1.34 \times Hgb \times (SaO_2 - SvO_2) \times 10$$

In this case, with a cardiac output of 5 L/min, the DO_2 is 250 mL O_2/minute. Indexed for a typical body surface area of 1.7 m^2, the DO_2I is 147 mL O_2/min/m^2.

Using The DO_2 and VO_2 Together

Knowing the DO_2 or VO_2 in isolation is not particularly useful. The clinical question is whether the delivery is adequate to meet the body's consumption requirements. To answer this, the DO_2:VO_2 ratio is helpful. During periods of both rest and exercise, the DO_2:VO_2 ratio is maintained at approximately 4:1 to 5:1 by changes in the cardiac output. This provides a reserve of sorts—after all, it wouldn't be very useful from a survival perspective to only deliver as much oxygen as the body absolutely needs at any given time. This lack of a physiologic reserve would mean that a person would have no ability to withstand a sudden change in circumstances like having to sprint away from an attacker, or deal with a high fever or pulmonary embolism.

As seen in the following figure, the DO_2 can vary widely as the VO_2 remains constant. This reflects the aforementioned physiologic reserve. As the DO_2 declines, however, it can reach a point at which further drops in oxygen delivery cause a drop in consumption. This point is known in physiology as the hypoxic, or anaerobic, threshold. It is at this point that the reserve is exhausted and the consumption becomes supply-dependent. A patient at or below this point for a prolonged period will become severely acidotic and, in most cases, will not survive.

It would make sense that the anaerobic threshold would occur when the DO_2 equals the VO_2. Experimentally, however, it has been shown that the threshold is closer to the 2:1 mark, and is explained by the variable oxygen consumption of different organ systems. Cardiac output delivered to hair, teeth, and bones doesn't contribute much to meet the needs of the more vital organ systems.

DO2:VO2 Relationship

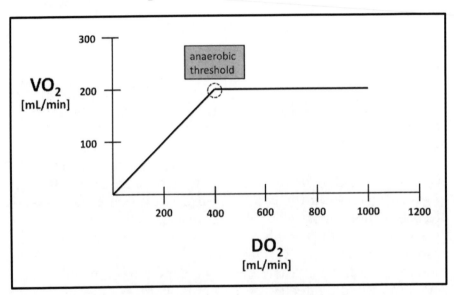

Mathematically, the DO_2:VO_2 ratio looks like this:

$$DO_2{:}VO_2 = \frac{CO \times 1.34 \times Hgb \times SaO_2 \times 10}{CO \times 1.34 \times Hgb \times (SaO_2 - SvO_2) \times 10}$$

Cancelling common factors greatly simplifies the equation:

$$DO_2:VO_2 = \frac{\cancel{CO} \times \cancel{1.34} \times \cancel{Hgb} \times SaO_2 \times \cancel{10}}{\cancel{CO} \times \cancel{1.34} \times \cancel{Hgb} \times (SaO_2 - SvO_2) \times \cancel{10}}$$

$$DO_2:VO_2 = \frac{SaO_2}{(SaO_2 - SvO_2)}$$

If the SaO_2 is assumed to be 100%, then the SvO_2 correlates with the $DO_2:VO_2$ ratio:

$DO_2:VO_2$	SvO_2
5:1	80%
4:1	75%
3:1	67%
2:1	50%

This correlation makes clinical estimation of the $DO_2:VO_2$ relationship much easier, as the SvO_2 can be measured directly and continuously by a pulmonary artery catheter. If a pulmonary artery catheter is not present, a central venous oxygen saturation ($ScvO_2$) can be measured by obtaining a venous blood gas from a central venous line placed in the internal jugular or subclavian vein. The $ScvO_2$ is usually 5-8% higher than the SvO_2. While not as accurate as the true mixed venous oxygen saturation obtained with a pulmonary artery catheter, the $ScvO_2$ can be used to estimate of the $DO_2:VO_2$ relationship.

The SvO_2, as a surrogate for the $DO_2:VO_2$ relationship, can be used to identify when a patient has insufficient oxygen delivery to meet consumption requirements. The SvO_2 also has the advantage of not requiring continuous calculation of the actual DO_2 and VO_2—any changes in the relationship between delivery and consumption will be reflected in the SvO_2. The SvO_2 drops as oxygen delivery drops relative to consumption. An SvO_2 below 70% should warrant evaluation, and an SvO_2 below 60% is definitely concerning—it means that the patient is approaching the anaerobic threshold.

Looking back at the DO_2 equation, impaired oxygen delivery is always due to either low cardiac output, anemia, or hypoxemia. Correction of these should increase DO_2, with a resultant increase in SvO_2. Keep in mind that the cardiac output has the most significant effect on DO_2, and conditions like congestive heart failure, hypovolemia, hemorrhagic shock, and cardiac tamponade will all reduce cardiac output. This leads us to the third rule of oxygen: *The SvO_2 is low in low-flow states.*

Using the SvO₂ With DO₂ and VO₂

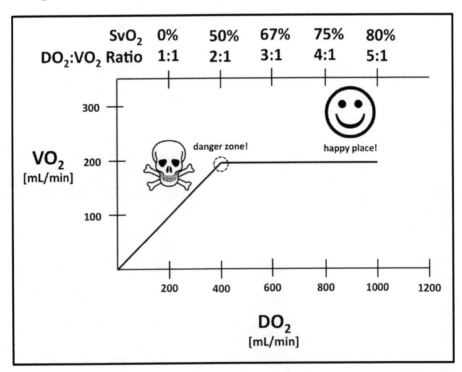

Patients with severe respiratory failure may have uncorrectable hypoxemia. A reduction in the SaO_2 will lead to a corresponding reduction in SvO_2 if the $DO_2{:}VO_2$ ratio remains constant. Calculating the oxygen extraction ratio is a quick way to estimate the balance between oxygen delivery and consumption even when the SaO_2 is markedly reduced:

$$O_2ER = \frac{SaO_2 - SvO_2}{SaO_2}$$

For a normal SaO_2 of 100% and SvO_2 of 75%, the O_2ER is: $(1.0 - 0.75)/1.0 = 0.25/1.0 = 0.25$, or 25%. This means that of the delivered oxygen, 25% was extracted and consumed by the tissues. A normal O_2ER is 20-25%.

As an example, consider a patient with severe respiratory failure whose SaO_2 is 84%. His SvO_2 is 60%. According to the above figure, an SvO_2 this low would be concerning. However, the assumption in Figure 2 is that the SaO_2 is 100%. Calculating the oxygen extraction ratio:

$O_2ER = (0.84 - 0.60)/0.84 = 0.24/0.84 = 0.286$, or 28.6%.

While this is a bit higher than the normal range of 20-25%, it isn't that much. Put another way, this indexing of the oxygen extraction would correlate with an SvO_2 of 71.4% (if the SaO_2 were 100%).

As a second example, take a patient with severe respiratory failure with an SaO_2 of 86%. His SvO_2 is 49%. The O_2ER is $(0.86 - 0.49)/0.86$, or 43%. This would correlate with an SvO_2 of 57% if the SaO_2 were 100%, and is certainly concerning for a low cardiac output state. An O_2ER of 30% or higher should warrant investigation, and an O_2ER higher than 40% indicates that the patient is approaching the anaerobic threshold.

The fourth rule of oxygen: *The DO_2:VO_2 ratio, SvO_2, and O_2ER reflect the balance between delivery and consumption. They don't represent a specific target for intervention.*

So, How Much Oxygen Is Really Needed?

Unfortunately for physiologists and writers of clinical algorithms, simply saying to keep the SvO_2 over 70% and all will be well doesn't work. This should come as no surprise to anyone familiar with the medical literature in critical care medicine—multiple studies proposing one physiologic manipulation or another have been consistently disproven. The combined processes of oxygen delivery, oxygen consumption, stress response, and cellular adaptation are far too complex to be summed up in this chapter, let alone a one-size-fits-all algorithm.

A normal PaO_2 while breathing ambient air at sea level is 90-100 mm Hg, but humans are able to tolerate much less over prolonged periods of time. The minimum necessary PaO_2 and SaO_2 is not known, and it is unlikely that any IRB will grant approval to a study aiming to withhold supplemental oxygen from critically ill patients. The degree of tolerable hypoxemia is also highly variable, and depends on factors such as the patient's age, comorbid conditions, living environment, genetic factors, and ability to cope with physiologic stress. What is known is that some people are able to survive moderate and even severe hypoxemia. Keep the following in mind:

- Mitochondrial PO_2 in cardiac and skeletal muscle is normally between 1 and 5 mm Hg.

- Oxidative phosphorylation in mitochondria doesn't begin to fail until the PO_2 is between 0.1 and 1 mm Hg.

- Climbers on Mount Everest who obtained femoral arterial samples from each other had PaO_2 in the 24-28 mm Hg range, and lived to tell the tale.

- In septic shock, the problem is not inadequate oxygen delivery. It's the inability of the tissues to properly metabolize the delivered oxygen. That's why patients die despite having an SvO_2 of 80%. The reasons for this are (very) incompletely understood.

- In the various ARDSNet trials, a PaO_2 as low as 55 mm Hg (with an SaO_2 of 88%) was considered acceptable. This is probably the best we will get as far as prospective evidence on the subject.

- Patients in the ARDSNet trial who received higher tidal volumes had better oxygenation, but also had a higher mortality rate. This suggests that preventing lung injury was more important than improving oxygenation.

- Many interventions have been shown to improve oxygenation in mechanically ventilated patients, but not to improve survival.

Using lactate levels is an appealing method of determining whether oxygen delivery is adequate, but it has its limitations as well. Most lactate production in critical illness is not due to anaerobic metabolism, despite common assumptions. Instead, it is a product of increased pyruvate production (with metabolism to lactate) in the setting of impaired or altered glycolysis and gluconeogenesis. Lactate is the preferred fuel for cardiac myocytes in the setting of adrenergic stimulation and is produced by aerobic cellular respiration. Thus, lactate should be viewed as a nonspecific marker of physiologic stress. If the lactate comes down following intubation, fluid resuscitation, etc., then it simply indicates that the patient is responding to therapy. It doesn't imply restoration of aerobic metabolism in previously anaerobic tissues. Likewise, an increasing lactate may indicate that the patient has a condition that is leading to an increase in sympathetic tone and cortisol-mediated stress response. Increasing oxygen delivery may or may not help the situation—it depends on what the underlying condition is.

This concept leads to the fifth rule of oxygen: *SaO_2, SvO_2, O_2ER, and lactate are all pieces of information and not goals in themselves.* They must be taken into account along with urine output, peripheral perfusion, mentation, and other clinical information before any treatment decisions can be made.

Oxygen Toxicity

The idea that supplemental oxygen can be toxic, especially in high doses, is not new. In neonates, high FiO_2 has been associated with retinopathy and bronchopulmonary dysplasia. In adults, there is evidence of worse outcomes with hyperoxia in the setting of acute myocardial infarction and following cardiac arrest. High FiO_2 in adults can cause irritation of the tracheobronchial tree and absorption atelectasis (due to the oxygen being absorbed without the stabilizing effect of nitrogen gas, leading to alveolar collapse).

Laboratory studies have demonstrated the increased presence of reactive oxygen species in the setting of infection, inflammation, and tissue reperfusion. The clinical significance of this is unclear, as the oxidative burst is a known component of inflammation and may be a part of the host response to infection. Reactive oxygen species can cause cellular injury and apoptosis *in vitro* but they rapidly combine with chloride and other ions *in vivo*, mitigating their effect. The degree to which the PaO_2 itself plays a role is also not fully understood, and it may be the case that the oxidative burst occurs as a part of inflammation or reperfusion under any kind of aerobic conditions (and not solely hyperoxic).

The degree to which clinically significant oxygen toxicity occurs in humans is poorly understood, and the role that the PaO_2 itself plays is unclear. Just because we don't know that there is toxicity, however, doesn't mean that it isn't occurring. The safest practice, then, is to treat oxygen like any other drug and to only give the patient as much as he needs. A useful analogy is the administration of norepinephrine in septic shock. A normal mean arterial pressure is 93 mm Hg, but organ perfusion is adequate with a mean arterial pressure of 65 mm Hg. Norepinephrine is titrated to achieve the lower target since that's all that's necessary. Aiming for the higher, "normal" target would require higher doses of norepinephrine and expose the patient to the risk of harm (ischemic fingers and toes, splanchnic vasoconstriction, increased afterload leading to impaired cardiac function, etc.).

Avoiding hyperoxia is easy, and can be accomplished by reducing the FiO_2. Even normoxia may not be necessary, and it may be prudent to tolerate a degree of permissive hypoxemia in order to avoid exposing the patient to high FiO_2 or ventilator pressures. Remember that cardiac output has a much more significant effect on oxygen delivery than the saturation, and focus on signs of adequate or inadequate oxygen delivery rather than strictly following the SaO_2 and PaO_2. This approach leads us to the sixth and final rule of oxygen: *Give the patient just as much oxygen as he needs. This may be less than you think.*

Six Rules Of Oxygen

1. The SaO_2 is what matters, not the PaO_2.

2. An increase in cardiac output can offset hypoxemia.

3. The SvO_2 is low in low-flow states

4. The DO_2:VO_2 ratio, SvO_2, and O_2ER reflect the balance between delivery and consumption. They don't represent a specific target for intervention.

5. SaO_2, SvO_2, O_2ER, and lactate are all pieces of information and not goals in themselves. They must be taken into account along with urine output, peripheral perfusion, mentation, and other clinical information before any treatment decisions can be made.

6. Give the patient just as much oxygen as he needs. This may be less than you think.

Chapter Two

Permissive Hypercapnia

Permissive hypercapnia is the practice of allowing a mechanically ventilated patient to develop or remain in a respiratory acidosis rather than exposing him to the risk of injurious ventilator settings. For the purposes of this chapter, permissive hypercapnia is defined as a $PaCO_2$ > 45 mm Hg with a pH < 7.35. Hickling et al. first described this concept in two papers that demonstrated a survival benefit with lower tidal volumes and elevated $PaCO_2$ levels.[1,2] This work was influential on later studies that showed the superiority of low tidal volume ventilation, including the landmark ARMA study performed by the ARDS Network investigators. Most of the studies examining this topic have focused on the benefit of using a lower tidal volume (4-6 mL/kg predicted body weight) in ARDS. There is less research on the benefits and risks of permissive hypercapnia itself, but there may be some advantages to permitting a mild to moderate respiratory acidosis in patients with severe respiratory failure.

Pulmonary Benefits of Permissive Hypercapnia

The primary rationale for hypercapnia is that avoiding iatrogenic ventilator-induced lung injury is more important that attaining normal gas exchange. Overdistension of healthy alveoli leads to cellular injury, and is referred to as volutrauma. This is the primary mechanism of ventilator-induced lung injury (VILI) and is independent of distending pressures (barotrauma). The ARMA study demonstrated a reduction in mortality in patients with ARDS when tidal volumes of 4-6 mL/kg PBW were used, compared with tidal volumes of 12 mL/kg.[3] This benefit was seen despite worsening gas exchange in the low tidal volume group. In patients with status asthmaticus, using lower tidal volumes and respiratory rates prevents dynamic hyperinflation, pneumothorax, and pneumomediastinum, even though it may lead to a respiratory acidosis. Permissive hypercapnia is considered acceptable because the benefits of avoiding lung injury are considered far more important than achieving "normal" alveolar ventilation.

Since current practice emphasizes the use of a low tidal volume in ARDS, increasing the tidal volume to correct a respiratory acidosis is seldom done. Instead, the respiratory rate is adjusted to increase or decrease the minute ventilation. Most of the time, increasing the respiratory rate on the ventilator is sufficient to blow off CO_2 and normalize the pH. This may not be necessary, however, as patients are able to tolerate even a significant respiratory acidosis so long as oxygenation is maintained.[4] In fact, there may be harm with this common practice. An increase in the frequency of tidal ventilation invariably leads to an increase in the cyclical opening and closure of vulnerable lung units. A patient with a set respiratory rate of 20 breaths per minute will have 11,520 more ventilatory cycles per day than another patient with a respiratory rate of 12 breaths per minute. Each one of those ventilatory cycles has the potential, albeit small, to contribute to VILI. Laboratory data supports the idea of using a lower ventilator rate whenever possible;[5] however, prospective studies in humans will be needed to validate this concept. In the absence of data, though, it is certainly reasonable to question the necessity of routinely increasing the ventilator rate to correct mild to moderate acidemia.

Extrapulmonary Benefits of Permissive Hypercapnia

No prospective, randomized human trials examining the extrapulmonary benefits of permissive hypercapnia have been done. There are several laboratory studies in animals that have demonstrated a beneficial effect of hypercapnia on free radical production, myocardial injury, and cerebral ischemia.[6] This reduction in pro-inflammatory cytokines and oxidative injury may prove to be helpful in reducing multisystem organ dysfunction, especially because the majority of patients with ARDS die of multisystem organ failure rather than of primary respiratory failure.

In healthy human volunteers, controlled hypercapnia under general anesthesia was shown to increase both cardiac output and tissue oxygenation.[7] A study of patients with severe ARDS demonstrated an increase in cardiac output and systemic oxygen delivery with a tidal volume reduction and hypercapnic acidosis;[8] the same study, however, also showed worsening right ventricular function and hemodynamics. In a study of patients with subarachnoid hemorrhage and cerebral vasospasm, controlled hypercapnia led to an increase in cerebral blood flow without prohibitory elevations in intracranial pressure.[9] While this is not sufficient to justify a change in recommended ventilator management, these findings do argue against the presumption of harm with respiratory acidosis during mechanical ventilation.

Buffering

In the ARMA study and subsequent ARDS Network studies, administration of buffering fluids was permitted to keep the pH ≥ 7.15. Sodium bicarbonate ($NaHCO_3$) is often used to treat acidemia, but it does have several drawbacks. Under usual conditions, the bicarbonate anion is converted to CO_2 and H_2O via carbonic anhydrase:

$$CO_2 + H_2O \leftrightarrow H_2CO_3 \leftrightarrow H^+ + HCO_3^-$$

The elimination of the excess CO_2 produced by this reaction is not normally an issue—one or two breaths are sufficient to clear it. In the setting of severe respiratory failure, however, elimination of the CO_2 may not be possible and the pH may in fact fall with the administration of sodium bicarbonate. In addition, CO_2 diffuses freely over cell membranes (including in the CSF), but HCO_3^- does not. This has the effect of worsening intracellular acidosis, even if the systemic pH rises. A transient hemodynamic improvement is often seen when a bolus of sodium bicarbonate (e.g., an "amp") is given, but this is more likely due to the loading of sodium than the change in pH— similar effects are seen with bolus dosing of hypertonic saline. Keep in mind that the $NaHCO_3$ given in a 50 mL ampule is 8.4%, which is a very hypertonic sodium solution.

THAM (tris-hydroxymethyl aminomethane) is a direct H^+ ion buffer that does not depend on alveolar ventilation like $NaHCO_3$. It also crosses cell membranes freely and produces intracellular buffering. This may be a more effective buffer for hypercapnic acidosis, but there are scant clinical data for its efficacy. At the time of this writing, the point is moot—THAM has been discontinued by the only manufacturer that was producing it.

The necessity for buffering a respiratory acidosis during mechanical ventilation is debatable. The purported benefits of permissive hypercapnia (beyond the prevention of volutrauma) may be lost when the pH is increased. Administration of sodium bicarbonate may have some adverse effects, as described above, and there are no available non-bicarbonate buffers available for clinical use. Additionally, acidemia may confer a protective effect on hepatic and renal function, and systemic acidosis shifts the oxygen-hemoglobin dissociation curve rightward, thereby augmenting tissue oxygen delivery. Using buffer therapy to keep the pH ≥ 7.15 is a common, but unproven, practice. Until clinical studies show a benefit to doing this, it would be prudent to reserve buffering for situations where the clinician feels that the acidosis is having an adverse effect on the patient.

Downsides of Permissive Hypercapnia

Despite the aforementioned benefits, there are some clinical downsides of hypercapnic acidosis in critically ill patients. The most widely recognized is the correlation between hypercapnia and intracranial hypertension. Hypercapnia does lead to vasodilatation, including cerebral vasodilatation. While this may augment cerebral oxygen delivery,[9] it also increases the intracerebral blood volume. If intracranial compliance is diminished, this can lead to higher intracranial pressure. This may or may not be dangerous, depending on the degree of intracranial hypertension, but it certainly bears consideration. If hypercapnia is unavoidable in a patient with significant brain injury, then intracranial pressure monitoring should be considered.

In patients with both acute and chronic pulmonary hypertension, hypercapnia can cause higher pulmonary artery pressures and lead to right ventricular dysfunction. Much of this is due to the underlying lung disease, but if there is clinical evidence of impaired hemodynamic function, then lowering the $PaCO_2$ may be beneficial.

Other systemic effects of hypercapnia are more related to the resulting acidosis than from the effect of the $PaCO_2$ itself.

21

These include impaired cardiac contractility, prolonged QT interval, decreased systemic vascular resistance, and hyperkalemia. If these occur, then buffer therapy may be warranted if other methods of correcting the respiratory acidosis would result in lung injury.

On a microcellular level, hypercapnia has been associated with increased tissue nitration and the production of peroxynitrite. This radical is released during conditions of physiologic stress, and may mediate tissue damage.[10] The significance of this in clinical medicine is yet to be determined. Neutrophilic activity against bacterial infection is also attenuated with hypercapnia, but this can be overcome with the administration of antibiotics.[11]

Summary and Recommendations

Permissive hypercapnia is a proven strategy for reducing VILI in patients with severe respiratory failure, be it due to ARDS or obstructive diseases like asthma or COPD. To state it simply, it's more important to prevent iatrogenic lung injury than to get "normal" gas exchange. The degree to which permissive hypercapnia has a clinical benefit beyond preventing volutrauma remains to be seen, but the existing literature suggests that this may be the case.

Takeaway Points Regarding Permissive Hypercapnia

- Pay attention to tidal volumes. For ARDS, 4-6 mL/kg PBW is recommended. For obstructive airway diseases, 6-8 mL/kg PBW is recommended. Exceeding these thresholds may increase the risk of VILI.

- High respiratory rates may bring the pH up and the $PaCO_2$ down, but this may be harmful due to repetitive cycling of vulnerable lung units.

- Acidemia in itself may be beneficial in critical illness by augmenting blood flow and tissue oxygen delivery.

- Look beyond the pH—consider buffer therapy, high respiratory rates, and alternative ventilator strategies only if the acidosis seems to be causing problems like intracranial hypertension, pulmonary hypertension, impaired cardiac contractility, refractory hyperkalemia, and systemic hypotension.

Chapter Three

Seven Rules For
Severe Respiratory Failure

Positive Pressure Ventilation is supportive, and may be therapeutic, but it is not curative.

Without mechanical ventilation, patients with severe respiratory failure will undoubtedly die. Positive pressure ventilation can reduce shunt, improve gas exchange, and take over the work of breathing until the patient has recovered. That doesn't mean, however, that the ventilator can do anything to reverse the underlying condition or disease process that has led to respiratory failure.

"It is incident to physicians, I am afraid, beyond all other men, to mistake subsequence for consequence."
    —Dr. Samuel Johnson

TWO

Don't hurt the patient any more than you have to.

Ventilator-induced lung injury (VILI) has been recognized as a necessary evil since the advent of modern critical care medicine, and to altogether eliminate the risk of any lung injury from the ventilator is not realistic. That said, much VILI is actually an unnecessary evil, since it occurs in the pursuit of "normal" gas exchange or "optimized" physiologic parameters. In cases of severe respiratory failure, the risk of VILI is high and the potential for rewards is small—it isn't reasonable to injure the patient's lungs in order to increase the PaO_2 from 65 to 95, when 65 is sufficient to maintain life. Focusing on doing the minimum intervention necessary to support the patient is much more likely to be helpful in the long run.

"As to diseases, make a habit of two things—to help, or at least, to do no harm."
    —Hippocrates

THREE

Throw normal values out the window.

Do what's necessary, not whatever is possible. Chasing the ideal of "normal" gas exchange will inevitably lead to VILI and unnecessary therapeutic interventions, all of which carry very real (and unwanted) side effects. With severe respiratory failure in particular, the twin objectives are to sustain the patient and minimize the risk of further injury. Sustaining the patient is obviously the more important objective, and there will be times when very high ventilator pressures are necessary to achieve it; however, anything that exposes the patient to real or potential harm should be justifiable.

As an aside, this can be the most difficult part of taking care of critically ill patients. We have all been taught what's "normal," and we all face the temptation to do things in order to bring things [lab values, physiologic measurements, vital signs] back into these ranges.

"Preconceived, fixed notions can be more damaging than cannon."
—*Barbara Tuchman*

Don't be afraid to experiment....

We use clinical studies and guidelines as a framework for therapy, but what works for one patient may not necessarily work for another. Additionally, the volume of evidence for the critical care of the most severely injured or ill patients is scant. Therefore, it takes a willingness to try different things and an ability to admit when a particular therapy isn't working. In these cases, protocols and clinical pathways can be harmful in that they can constrain physicians from trying a new approach to the problem.

"Most of our assumptions have outlived their uselessness."
—*Marshall McLuhan*

... But don't be afraid to stay the course.

Trying a different approach may be necessary. More often than not, however, the patient is adequately sustained with his current ventilator settings but the clinicians are tempted to change course in order to improve the numbers. This has the potential for harm without much benefit and should be avoided. Any modifications should be done either to lower the risk of injury or if the current settings are not providing an acceptable degree of life support. Keep in mind that the medical literature is full of therapies that improve oxygenation, ventilation, and vital signs. Very few of these have actually translated into better patient outcomes.

"Difficulties are just things to overcome, after all."
    —Ernest Shackleton

Tracheotomize early.

Patients with severe respiratory failure are in it for the long haul. This means that the chances of improvement in a few days are low and that the need for at least some mechanical ventilator support for several weeks or months is quite high. Couple this with the sedation requirements and relative immobility that accompanies endotracheal intubation, and it's obvious that the sooner the patient has a tracheostomy, the sooner he can begin some degree of mobilization and rehabilitation. A tracheostomy is associated with less sedation, more patient comfort, better mobilization, and fewer days on the ventilator when compared with the endotracheal tube. Do it as soon as it's safe.

"You were sick, but now you're well again, and there's work to do."
    —Kurt Vonnegut

SEVEN

Remain positive.

Most patients with respiratory failure, even severe ARDS, will eventually recover. Those who survive ARDS will have near-normal lung function after six to twelve months. Even people with cardiopulmonary or neurologic disease who ultimately require a long-term tracheostomy can have an acceptable quality of life. Declaring a patient "ventilator-dependent" or saying that he has "no chance of recovery" after one or two weeks in the ICU may be premature or even wrong. Unbridled optimism isn't appropriate, but neither is pessimistic nihilism.

Some conditions are not survivable. Some conditions are survivable, and even have the potential for some recovery, but will leave the patient with significant disability and the need for partial or full ventilatory support. Lastly, some conditions are survivable and will require a prolonged period of critical care and ventilatory support, but with a chance at a full recovery to independence. Obviously, nothing is guaranteed, but clinicians caring for patients with respiratory failure should be able to discern which scenario is most likely and present this to the patient and his family.

Once a treatment plan is decided upon, it is imperative for the clinician to maintain a positive outlook. The patient and his family will be looking for encouragement and guidance, especially when there's a setback or a run of bad days. Throughout the course, the most important thing is open and honest communication. There are times when a shift to palliative care or hospice is appropriate—failure to recover, development of a new and severe complication, or if the patient is unwilling to continue a therapy with a small chance of success that is associated with significant discomfort or an unacceptable quality of life. In these situations, providing the patient and his family with a peaceful, comfortable death is a vital function of the clinician. There may be other times, however, when a setback is temporary and reversible, albeit discouraging (for example, development of pneumonia that requires going back to full ventilator support until it's adequately treated). Here, the clinician should encourage the patient and continue to focus on the ultimate goal of therapy, which is recovery to an acceptable quality of life.

"Attitude is a little thing that makes a big difference."
    —*Winston Churchill*

Chapter Four

PEEP, More PEEP, and Optimal PEEP

Positive end-expiratory pressure (PEEP) is used during mechanical ventilation to maintain alveolar patency and to improve oxygenation. When the ventilator delivers a breath, the airway pressure is raised to the peak airway pressure (or peak inspiratory pressure). Expiration is passive, but instead of allowing the lungs to exhale until the pressure is atmospheric (i.e., zero), the ventilator stops expiratory flow when the pressure reaches the preset end-expiratory pressure. This is analogous to breathing out while a large fan blows air into your lungs—it provides a pressurized splint of air, which in turn maintains airway and alveolar patency when they would otherwise collapse. During conventional mechanical ventilation, this is known as PEEP. During spontaneous and noninvasive ventilation, it is called continuous positive airway pressure (CPAP). Since both have the same physiologic effect, they are essentially synonymous.

PEEP is most often applied and adjusted to improve a patient's oxygenation. The primary effect of PEEP in hypoxemic respiratory failure is to reduce the fraction of intrapulmonary shunting; that is, areas of the lungs that are perfused but not ventilated. The more alveolar flooding there is (from pulmonary edema, bleeding, pneumonia, exudate, etc.), the more pressure is needed to open up collapsed lung units. The patient's chest X-ray can be used as a rough guide for the initial PEEP.

Initial PEEP Settings in the Emergency Department or ICU

Chest X-Ray	Initial PEEP
Clear	5 cm H_2O
Scattered Infiltrates	10 cm H_2O
Diffuse Dense Infiltrates	15 cm H_2O
Bilateral White Out	20 cm H_2O

The majority of patients with hypoxemic respiratory failure can be managed rather easily with a PEEP in the range of 5-10 cm H_2O. In those with moderate to severe acute respiratory distress syndrome (ARDS), a more intensive regimen may be required. This is known as trying to set the "best PEEP" or "optimal PEEP"—that is, the PEEP that attains the best oxygenation and compliance while minimizing the risk of ventilator-induced lung injury. Numerous clinical approaches to the problem of finding the "optimal PEEP" for a patient have been described in the medical literature, and each method has both adherents and detractors. As you might expect, each method has its strong points and drawbacks, and no one approach is superior to the rest (otherwise everyone would use it and ignore the others). These will be discussed in turn.

ARDSNet Tables

The tables used in the ARDSNet studies have the advantage of simplicity and titratability to oxygenation, which can be measured easily with an arterial blood gas or a pulse oximeter. Two tables have been published—one that uses a high-PEEP approach, and one using lower levels of PEEP. The two methods were compared head-to-head in the ALVEOLI study,[12] which did not demonstrate improved outcomes from either approach as long as a lung-protective tidal volume of 4-6 mL/kg PBW was used. This is actually advantageous to the physician— it suggests that either table can be used, depending on the patient's condition. A patient who is morbidly obese, or who has abdominal compartment syndrome, has reduced chest wall compliance and might benefit from a higher-PEEP strategy. The extrinsic compression of the lungs, combined with the poor lung compliance due to ARDS, means that a higher expiratory pressure should be used to prevent alveolar collapse and derecruitment.

On the other hand, using a lower level of PEEP might be indicated in some cases. A patient with a bronchopleural fistula, or one with tenuous hemodynamics, or someone with one lung significantly more injured than the other, may get worse with a high-PEEP strategy. Since one table doesn't have any proven advantage over the other, the physician can pick whichever one seems to fit the patient better.

Using the ARDSNet PEEP Tables

- PEEP is measured in cm H_2O
- Go up and down the table as needed to keep the PaO_2 55-80 mm Hg, or the SpO_2 88-94%

Lower PEEP Table

FiO₂	PEEP
30%	5
40%	5
40%	8
50%	8
50%	10
60%	10
70%	10
70%	12
70%	14
80%	14
90%	14
90%	16
90%	18
100%	18
100%	20
100%	22
100%	24

Higher PEEP Table

FiO₂	PEEP
30%	5
30%	8
30%	10
30%	12
30%	14
40%	14
40%	16
50%	16
50%	18
50%	20
60%	20
70%	20
80%	20
80%	22
90%	22
100%	22
100%	24

Decremental PEEP Trial

The method of the decremental PEEP trial is that the patient's lungs should be recruited as fully as possible using a CPAP recruitment maneuver, followed by a stepwise gradual reduction in expiratory pressure until there is a drop-off in oxygenation, or compliance, or both. This has the advantage of being easy to perform at the bedside; additionally, monitoring oxygenation is easily done with a pulse oximeter, and most ventilators will display static and dynamic respiratory system compliance.*

A decremental PEEP trial is performed as follows. Remember that you are going to **Recruit, Reduce,** and **Recruit.**

- Ensure the patient is adequately sedated. Neuromuscular blockade is not necessary as long as the patient isn't making a lot of spontaneous respiratory effort.

- Set the ventilator to an FiO_2 of 100%.

- Put the ventilator on CPAP 40 cm H_2O, with no pressure support. Hold at this level for 40 seconds (40 for 40). This is the recruitment maneuver.

- After the recruitment maneuver, change the ventilator mode to either Volume Control with a tidal volume of 6 mL/kg PBW, or Pressure Control with a driving pressure of 15 cm H_2O. Set the PEEP at 20 cm. Note the patient's compliance.

---

* Compliance = ΔVolume / ΔPressure

Dynamic compliance on the ventilator =
Tidal Volume / [Peak Inspiratory Pressure − PEEP]

Static compliance on the ventilator = Tidal Volume / [Plateau Pressure − PEEP]

- Reduce the FiO_2 by 10-20% at a time every 5-10 minutes until the SpO_2 levels off at 88-94%.

- Once the FiO_2 has been reduced, begin dropping the PEEP in 2 cm increments every 5-10 minutes until the SpO_2 falls below 88%, or until there's a notable drop in compliance. Either of these would indicate alveolar derecruitment.

- Repeat the recruitment maneuver (40 for 40), and set the PEEP at 2 cm higher than the level where derecruitment occurred.

The disadvantages of a decremental PEEP trial include the time required to properly perform the trial, the need for deep sedation, and the possibility of hemodynamic or respiratory compromise during the recruitment maneuver. Clinical trials examining the decremental PEEP strategy have found that it may improve oxygenation and respiratory compliance, but have not proven any benefit toward survival. It may not be reasonable to perform a trial on every ventilated patient in the ICU. For those with moderate to severe ARDS, however, this can be a useful tool for finding an appropriate level of PEEP.

Pressure-Volume Curves

Using a dynamic pressure-volume loop to determine the optimal level of PEEP is appealing. Many ventilators can produce the P-V loop for review, and it seems intuitive that setting the PEEP at or above the point where pulmonary compliance falls would be useful.

The inspiratory limb of the P-V curve is thought to represent the change in compliance as the lungs fill with gas. Initially, the compliance (the slope of the curve) is poor, reflecting the significant inspiratory pressure needed to open collapsed lung units. Once these lung units open up, they inflate rapidly and much more easily. This is the steeper part of the inspiratory P-V curve, and it indicates that the compliance of the respiratory system has improved. The point where the compliance changes (in other words, where the slope of the curve changes) is known as the lower inflection point (LIP).

As the lungs continue to fill with gas, they reach a point where further application of pressure doesn't expand the lungs much at all—this occurs at the upper inflection point (UIP), and inspiratory pressures beyond this point are thought to contribute to alveolar overdistension and potential barotrauma.

Upper and Lower Inflection Points

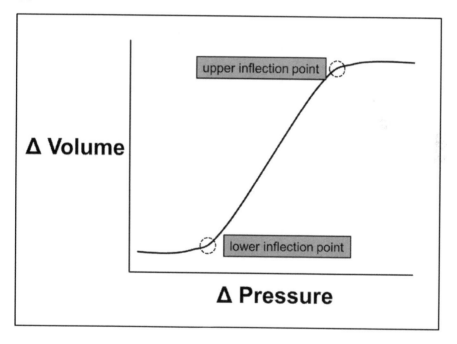

Theoretically, using the inspiratory P-V curve should tell the clinician everything he needs to know regarding the PEEP and driving pressure. The PEEP should be set at or just above the lower inflection point to keep the alveoli from collapsing during expiration, and the plateau pressure (that is, the alveolar pressure at end-inspiration) should be kept at or just below the upper inflection point to minimize overdistension and barotrauma. This would keep the patient ventilating along the steep part of the compliance curve.

Unfortunately, it's not that easy. To begin with, establishing a true pressure-volume curve is difficult. The patient can't be breathing spontaneously, because patient-initiated breathing alters intra- and extrathoracic mechanics. Neuromuscular blockade and deep sedation are often necessary. Second, the inspiratory flow must be constant and relatively low—using a decelerating inspiratory flow, which is the case in pressure control ventilation and pressure-regulated volume control ventilation, will produce an inaccurate curve. Third, the PEEP must be at zero during the maneuver, which can be risky in a severely hypoxemic patient. Fourth, and perhaps most important, is the argument that it makes little sense to set an expiratory pressure based on inspiratory pulmonary mechanics.

Clinical data in humans has shown that while there is some rationale for the lower inflection point, alveolar recruitment tends to continue during the entire inspiratory cycle. Additionally, the upper inflection point may represent the end of the recruitment process but not necessarily alveolar overdistension. During expiration, which is largely passive, an expiratory inflection point occurs at a pressure much higher than the inspiratory lower inflection point. This would suggest that alveolar derecruitment begins at a much higher pressure than the LIP, and that in ARDS this may be as high as 20-22 cm H_2O.[13] Additionally, derecruitment is affected by gravity and the position of the patient. The heterogeneous nature of both ARDS and alveolar recruitment/derecruitment makes the use of a single pressure-volume relationship difficult when it comes to setting the PEEP.

Inspiratory and Expiratory Inflection Points

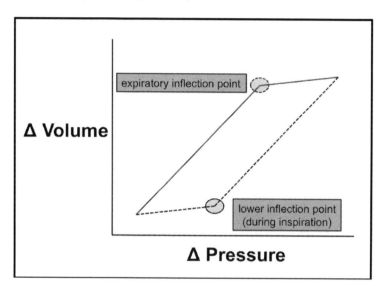

PEEP At Different Inflection Points

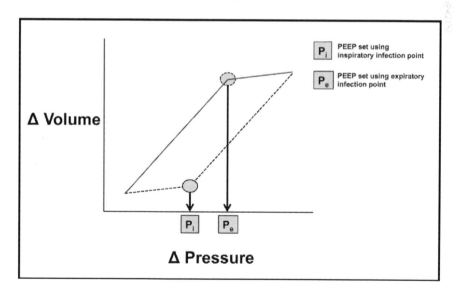

Plateau Pressure-Guided Titration

The plateau pressure (P_{PLAT}) is the pressure measured at the end of inspiration when inspiratory flow is held at zero. This pressure reflects equilibration of pressures throughout the respiratory tree, and presumably is the end-inspiratory alveolar pressure. In general, clinicians should aim to keep the plateau pressure less than 30-35 cm H_2O, as this is felt to be the upper limit of alveolar pressure before lung injury occurs*. In the ExPress trial, the tidal volume was set at 6 mL/kg predicted body weight, and the PEEP was increased until the P_{PLAT} was 28-30 cm H_2O.[14] The control group had a PEEP of 5-9 cm H_2O. The hypothesis was that this would lead to full alveolar recruitment while preventing lung injury. The trial did demonstrate an improvement in oxygenation in the group receiving this intervention; however, there was no difference in survival.

One drawback of this approach is that patients with less severe ARDS may actually receive higher levels of PEEP. Take two patients with ARDS who each have a predicted body weight of 67 kg. For both, the tidal volume should be 400 mL. If one has less severe ARDS and a respiratory system compliance of 40 mL/cm H_2O, then it will take an inspiratory driving pressure of 10 cm to deliver the tidal volume. Addition of 18 cm PEEP would bring the plateau pressure up to 28.

In the case of the second patient, assume that his condition is worse and that his respiratory compliance is 20 mL/cm H_2O. This requires a driving pressure of 20 cm to get the tidal volume, and by following this protocol, he would only get 8-10 cm PEEP to bring the P_{PLAT} up to 28-30.

---

* It is important to keep in mind that no one has established a truly "safe" level of plateau pressure, above which lung injury is present and below which no injury occurs. Most experts, however, advise keeping the plateau pressure at or below this range.

This example is simplistic and purposefully ignores the fact that compliance would change (for either better or worse) with the application of PEEP, but the point is that targeting one specific number in all patients could be harmful. It is also worth considering that this method of setting PEEP did not improve survival when compared with the control group.

Transpulmonary Pressure

The transmural, or transpulmonary, pressure in the lung is defined as the difference between the pressure inside the alveoli and the pleural pressure. In other words, Pressure (in) – Pressure (out). Under normal conditions, this value is quite small—the alveolar pressure is atmospheric, or zero, while breathing through an open glottis, and the pleural pressure ranges from around -3 cm H_2O at end-expiration to -8 cm at end-inspiration. Since the transpulmonary pressure is the difference between the two, it ranges from 3 (0 - -3) to 8 (0 - -8) cm H_2O. This is what keeps the lungs open and acts as a counterbalance to the elastic recoil of the lung.

During positive pressure ventilation, the alveolar pressure becomes positive and ranges between the plateau pressure at end-inspiration and the end-expiratory pressure (PEEP). The pleural pressure, if unchanged, remains slightly negative. Under certain conditions, however, the pleural pressure may become positive. This usually occurs when there is a reduction in chest wall compliance either due to primary pleural disease or extrinsic compression (increased abdominal pressure, volume overload, morbid obesity, or a circumferential burn of the torso). When this occurs, the transpulmonary pressure is reduced.

Take two patients with ARDS who have a PEEP set at 15 cm. The first patient has no extrinsic chest wall restriction and a pleural pressure of -5 cm. His transpulmonary pressure at end-expiration is 20 (15 - ⁻5), which serves to maintain alveolar recruitment in the setting of lung inflammation and edema.

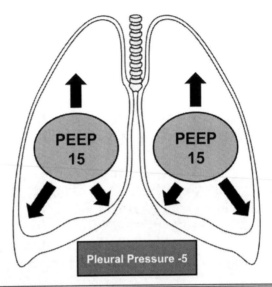

Transpulmonary Pressure = PEEP – Pleural Pressure

Transpulmonary Pressure = 15 – (-5) = 20

Net Pressure Effect Leads To Alveolar Expansion

The second patient, in addition to having ARDS, also has reduced chest wall compliance due to morbid obesity (BMI 52). His pleural pressure is +18 cm, which means that his transpulmonary pressure at end-expiration is -3 (15 - ⁺18). The net effect is alveolar collapse at the end of each respiratory cycle.

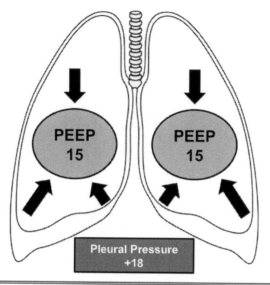

Direct measurement of the intrapleural pressure in ICU patients isn't possible, so the esophageal pressure is used as a surrogate. This is by no means exact—pleural pressure itself varies from the base of the lung to the apex and is affected by supine or prone positioning, and esophageal pressure is subjected to the weight of the mediastinal contents.[15] It is, however, useful for titrating PEEP in patients in whom there is considerable extrinsic reduction of chest compliance.

In order to measure esophageal pressure (P_{eso}), an air-filled esophageal balloon catheter must be inserted. These are commercially available[16] and can be connected to a standard pressure monitoring system. The CareFusion Avea® ventilator has a port to connect an esophageal pressure probe and can display the esophageal pressure as well.

Insertion of the esophageal balloon catheter should be done by a qualified practitioner in accordance with the manufacturer's instructions. The depth to which the catheter should be inserted can be estimated by multiplying the patient's height in centimeters by 0.288. This should, in most people, position the balloon in the lower third of the esophagus. Partial inflation of the balloon with 1 mL of air will allow changes in the esophageal pressure to be reflected on the monitor. The esophageal pressure waveform should slightly increase during ventilator-delivered breaths and have a negative deflection during patient-initiated breaths. Gentle pressure applied to the abdomen that leads to an increase in the pressure reading suggests gastric placement of the balloon, and it should be withdrawn.

Once the esophageal balloon catheter is in proper position, the end-expiratory transpulmonary pressure can be calculated:

Transpulmonary Pressure = PEEP − [P_{eso} − 5][*]

For a patient with a PEEP of 15 cm and a P_{ESO} of 22, his end-expiratory transpulmonary pressure is -2 cm H_2O. In other words, at end expiration the compression of his lungs by the increased pleural pressure is leading to alveolar collapse. In this situation, the PEEP should be increased to a minimum level of 17 to keep the end-expiratory transpulmonary pressure at zero.

---

[*] 5 cm is subtracted from the P_{eso} to account for mediastinal weight. This is a crude estimation, not an exact measurement.

One clinical trial examining the effect of transpulmonary pressure monitoring in patients with ARDS demonstrated a significant improvement in oxygenation but did not show a survival benefit.[17] As such, this technique is not recommended for routine use. It may be helpful, though, in determining the appropriate level of PEEP for patients with intra-abdominal hypertension or morbid obesity.

Optimal PEEP vs. Good Enough PEEP

In a trial of 51 patients with ARDS, Chiumello and colleagues examined different methods of setting PEEP (ARDSNet tables, targeting a plateau pressure a la the ExPress trial, using the time-pressure stress index, and via transpulmonary pressure using esophageal pressure measurement).[18] All methods were assessed using CT scanning to determine the change in recruitability of the lung. Their findings suggested that the only method that correlated with the degree of whole-lung recruitability and the severity of ARDS was the use of the PEEP-FiO2 table. The other methods were associated with more hyperexpansion of normal lung units without a commensurate benefit in recruitment of collapsed alveoli.

The multiple methods of determining the best, or optimal, level of PEEP have a few things in common. They tend to be laborious. They tend to make significant physiologic assumptions that may not be valid—for example, the assumption that the pressure in the lower esophagus accurately reflects pleural pressure throughout the patient, or the assumption that lung recruitment is complete by the lower inflection point of the inspiratory pressure-volume curve. Lastly, they most often focus on surrogate endpoints that may not be meaningful. Clinical trials of different maneuvers designed to find optimal PEEP often report improved oxygenation or compliance when compared with controls, but none have shown a survival benefit.

Perhaps we need to stop searching for optimal PEEP. The history of critical care medicine has consistently shown that attempts by clinicians to optimize different physiologic parameters are often unnecessary and occasionally harmful.[*] This may be no different. Luciano Gattinoni, one of the foremost researchers in the field, has suggested this very thing. A "good enough" PEEP maintains oxygenation and lung recruitment without compromising hemodynamic function, and can be based on a combination of the severity of ARDS and the good sense of the treating clinician.

Good Enough PEEP[19]

Degree of ARDS	PaO$_2$/FiO$_2$ Ratio	PEEP
Mild	201-300	5-10 cm H$_2$O
Moderate	101-200	10-15 cm H$_2$O
Severe	≤ 100	15-20 cm H$_2$O

---

[*] Perioperative hemodynamic optimization using the pulmonary artery catheter; ScvO2 monitoring in septic shock; aggressive transfusion strategies in penetrating trauma, GI hemorrhage, and critical illness; decompressive craniectomy to treat intracranial hypertension; intra-aortic balloon counterpulsation for cardiogenic shock; high-frequency oscillatory ventilation for ARDS. The beat goes on....

Chapter Five

Severe Bronchospasm

Mechanical ventilation of patients with severe bronchospasm can be very difficult. This usually occurs with status asthmaticus, but it can also be seen with respiratory failure due to chronic obstructive lung disease, inhalation of toxic fumes, and viral bronchiolitis. Status asthmaticus in particular can be tough to treat due to the combination of bronchospasm and mucus plugging, which significantly worsens ventilation-perfusion matching.

Respiratory care of the patient with severe bronchospasm begins with treatment of the underlying condition. Asthma and COPD exacerbations are treated with inhaled beta-adrenergic agonists like albuterol; inhaled anti-muscarinics like ipratropium bromide; and systemic corticosteroids. The dosing of corticosteroids depends on the disease in question and the underlying pathophysiology. Asthma has a strong allergic component and is associated with inflammation and airway hyper-responsiveness. Initial dosing of corticosteroids in the ICU should be 1-2 mg/kg of prednisone (or equivalent) daily. The bronchospasm in COPD, on the other hand, is more related to excessive mucus production and narrowing of airways due to dynamic collapse during forced exhalation. It has much less of an inflammatory component when compared with asthma. Lower dosing of prednisone (or equivalent) is appropriate. Most studies suggest that there is little benefit from a prednisone dose in excess of 40-60 mg per day for COPD exacerbations, and there is always the potential for harmful effects from higher doses. Corticosteroids do not have a linear dose-response relationship in respiratory illness—doubling the steroid dose will not halve the bronchospasm.

For those patients with bronchospasm requiring mechanical ventilation, it is important to differentiate high airway resistance from high alveolar pressure. This can be done by performing an inspiratory pause maneuver on the ventilator. At the end of inspiration, flow is temporarily stopped for 0.5 to 1.0 seconds. During this time, pressures will equilibrate across the respiratory system. The pressure in the endotracheal tube will be the same (or nearly so) as the pressure in the alveoli. This is known as the plateau pressure (P_{PLAT}). The difference between the peak inspiratory pressure (PIP) and the P_{PLAT} is an estimate of the airway resistance. Normally, the gradient between the PIP and P_{PLAT} is 5 cm or less. If the gradient is higher, then the resistance to flow is elevated. This can be due to an issue with the endotracheal tube—if it's a small-diameter tube, or if it's kinked, or if it's partially plugged with mucus, the airway resistance will rise. If the tube is functioning well, is properly sized, and not obstructed, then a high airway resistance usually means that there's bronchospasm present (even if wheezing can't be auscultated). Treatment with inhaled beta-agonists and anti-muscarinics may help.

If the PIP and P_{PLAT} are both elevated, especially if the P_{PLAT} is over 30 cm H_2O, then it indicates increased alveolar pressure. Common situations that increase the alveolar pressure include mainstem intubation (all the volume for two lungs is going into one); pneumothorax; pulmonary edema; mucus plugging leading to atelectasis; dynamic hyperinflation; and increased abdominal pressure. While all of these can occur in any patient requiring mechanical ventilation, asthmatics are especially prone to mucus plugging, dynamic hyperinflation, and pneumothorax. These should definitely be considered in any ventilated asthmatic who suddenly gets worse.

Dynamic hyperinflation can be diagnosed both on the ventilator and by physical exam. On examination, the patient will usually appear uncomfortable. Paradoxical breathing, with the chest and abdomen moving in a dyssynchronous manner, can be seen. On auscultation, loud wheezing can be heard right up until the next breath is delivered. The cardiac monitor may display lower voltage of the QRS complex during inspiration, due to the trapped gas in the thorax impeding the electrical current. If the patient has an arterial line, pulsus paradoxus* may be present. The patient's jugular veins may be distended during expiration but collapse during inspiration, owing to the increased intrathoracic pressure at the end of expiration.

On the ventilator, dynamic hyperinflation can be observed by looking at the expiratory flow-time waveform. Normally, at end-expiration the flow should be zero. All of the gas has escaped, leaving the lungs at functional residual capacity. With dynamic hyperinflation, there is usually some expiratory gas flow ongoing at the time of the next inspiration. This may not always be present, however, and so an expiratory pause maneuver should be performed if dynamic hyperinflation is suspected.

---

* A drop in the systolic blood pressure by more than 10 mm Hg during inspiration. The "paradox" is that the heart is still beating, but the radial pulse may be absent. Pulsus paradoxus can also be seen with cardiac tamponade, constrictive pericarditis, anaphylaxis, pneumothorax, and other conditions.

Dynamic Hyperinflation

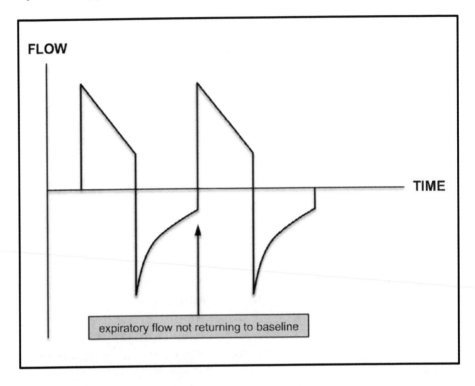

The mechanics behind the expiratory pause maneuver are similar to the inspiratory pause—when flow stops, pressure equilibrates. This time, the pressure is equilibrating at the end of expiration, when alveolar pressure should normally be zero. If any PEEP is set on the ventilator, the alveolar pressure should equal the PEEP. With dynamic hyperinflation, the actual (or measured) end-expiratory pressure will be higher than the applied (or set) PEEP. This is why dynamic hyperinflation is often referred to as "auto-PEEP."

Expiratory Pause Maneuver Demonstrating Auto-PEEP

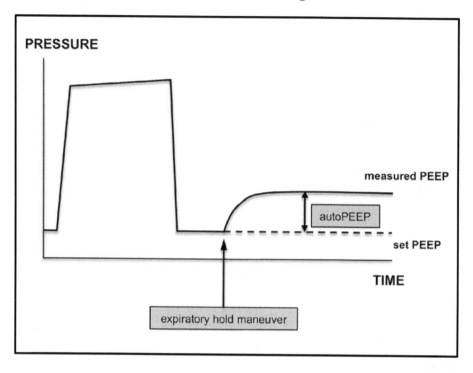

Ventilator Management

The goals with mechanical ventilation in the patient with severe bronchospasm are to minimize hyperinflation, allow the respiratory muscles to rest, and to avoid complications like pneumothorax, pneumomediastinum, and pulmonary interstitial emphysema. With regard to gas exchange, the goal is adequate (not perfect) oxygenation and toleration of hypercapnic acidosis.

Dynamic hyperinflation can be minimized by simply giving the patient enough time to exhale completely. This can be done by lowering the respiratory rate and/or reducing the inspiratory time (the time it takes for the breath to be delivered). Of the two, lowering the respiratory rate is the most effective. Consider a patient with a respiratory rate of 20 and an inspiratory time (I-time) of 1 second. With 20 breaths per minute, there are 3 seconds allocated per breath. The I-time is set at 1.0 seconds, leaving 2.0 seconds for expiration. The ratio between inspiration and expiration time is thus 1:2. If the clinician wants to permit more time for expiration, he can shorten the inspiratory time and prolong the I:E ratio. In this example, if the I-time is lowered to 0.7 seconds, there are now 2.3 seconds left for expiration. This translates to an I:E ratio of 1:3.3. This is better, but it may not be sufficient to permit adequate expiration through narrowed, inflamed airways. You will also find that shortening the inspiratory time by too much can cause a good bit of air hunger and discomfort, as well as very high peak inspiratory pressures. In turn, this can lead to heavy sedation and neuromuscular blockade. Try taking in your breaths in 0.5 seconds—you won't like it for long.

Lowering the respiratory rate is the more effective way of prolonging the I:E ratio while minimizing patient discomfort. In the example above, if we lower the respiratory rate to 15, there are now 4 seconds per breath. If the I-time is kept at 1.0 second, the expiratory time is 3.0 seconds. The I:E ratio is 1:3. Lower the respiratory rate to 12, and the I:E ratio is 1:4. A rate of 10—the I:E ratio is 1:5. Most of the time, there isn't much benefit to an I:E ratio any longer than 1:5.

Low tidal volumes can also work against the patient with severe bronchospasm, especially if he isn't heavily sedated. Air hunger is a common symptom of an exacerbation of asthma or COPD, and low tidal volumes can make the patient very tachypneic. A tidal volume of 6 mL/kg predicted body weight (PBW) is great for ARDS, but with asthma and COPD, a higher tidal volume is often needed. 8 mL/kg PBW usually works without causing overdistension, and it mitigates the tachypnea and air hunger. Higher tidal volumes, especially > 10 mL/kg PBW, do increase the risk of barotrauma.

Adequate sedation and analgesia is important. The discomfort of the endotracheal tube, along with the tachypnea associated with an exacerbation of pulmonary disease, can lead to air trapping and hyperinflation. Narcotic analgesia (like a fentanyl infusion) minimizes the discomfort of the tube and other devices and helps take away the subjective feeling of breathlessness. Titratable sedatives such as propofol and dexmetetomidine may also be helpful. Use of a sedation scale, such as the Richmond Agitation-Sedation Scale (RASS), is important for nursing staff to titrate the sedation. In my experience, titration to a RASS of -1 to -2 is effective in patients with severe bronchospasm. Neuromuscular blockade can be used if the patient-ventilator dyssynchrony is severe or if the dynamic hyperinflation is causing significant hemodynamic instability. It should be used sparingly and only until the patient stabilizes, however, due to the higher risk of critical illness-associated weakness with these drugs (especially when corticosteroids are also administered, as they usually are). Of the neuromuscular blockers available, cistatracurium is preferred due to its metabolism not being affected by renal or hepatic dysfunction.

> **Initial Ventilator Settings for Severe Bronchospasm**
>
> - **Mode: Assist-Control Ventilation**
> - **Rate: 10-14 Breaths/minute**
> - **Adjust Inspiratory Time to keep I:E ratio 1:3—1:5**
> - **Constant inspiratory flow**
> - **Tidal Volume: 8 mL/kg PBW**
> - **PEEP: zero (or ZEEP)***
> - **FiO2: 100% to start, adjusted downward to keep SpO$_2$ 88-95%**

The concept of permissive hypercapnia is very important when caring for patients with severe bronchospasm. The idea is that preventing lung injury (in the form of dynamic hyperinflation or barotrauma) is more important than having normal gas exchange. Maintaining adequate oxygenation is important—keep the SpO$_2$ 88-95%, and the PaO$_2$ 55-80 mm Hg. The PaCO$_2$ is less important, unless there is a significant coexisting condition like increased intracranial pressure that precludes permissive hypercapnia. In general, as long as the pH is kept above 7.10, it's all right to allow the PaCO$_2$ to rise. Buffer therapy such as sodium bicarbonate infusions can also be used to keep the pH above this threshold. The adoption of permissive hypercapnia seems to be associated with a significant decline in the mortality seen with status asthmaticus and mechanical ventilation.[20]

---

* Alveolar flooding and collapse is usually not a problem with status asthmaticus or exacerbation of COPD. Applying PEEP, especially with status asthmaticus, can worsen air trapping and hyperinflation. There is occasionally a role for applied PEEP with dynamic airway collapse, like in a COPD exacerbation, but to start with I recommend zero end-expiratory pressure (ZEEP). This is discussed further in *The Ventilator Book*.

Most of the time, the measures described above are sufficient to treat the patient with severe bronchospasm. Keep the vent rate low; administer albuterol, ipratropium, and prednisone; don't stress about the $PaCO_2$; and let the patient get better. This usually works, until it doesn't. When the patient is still deteriorating, the clinician should consider one or more rescue therapies. These include Heliox, ketamine infusion, and therapeutic bronchoscopy. Inhalational anesthetics have been described in the literature, but the cumbersome nature of anesthesia machines and the potential toxicity of leaking anesthetic gases to hospital staff make this a less desirable option.

Heliox

Heliox refers to a blend of helium and oxygen, usually in a 70:30 ratio. A gas blender can be used to change this ratio to 60:40. When the fraction of oxygen exceeds 40%, the potential benefit of Heliox is lost. Therefore, Heliox should only be used when the patient can be adequately oxygenated with an FiO_2 of 40% or less.

The benefit of Heliox is with the helium having a much lower density than nitrogen gas. This translates into Heliox improving the tendency of inspired gas toward laminar flow, which improves gas flow through narrowed proximal and larger airways. More laminar and less turbulent gas flow in the conducting airways leads to better gas exchange and aerosol delivery of medications like albuterol to the respiratory and terminal bronchioles. This can also help reduce the work of breathing. Heliox can be delivered by facemask, through noninvasive positive pressure breathing, or via the mechanical ventilator.

Two issues must be addressed when using Heliox through the ventilator. The first is the mode of ventilation. Most newer ventilators are not calibrated for a mixture of helium and oxygen. The inspiratory valve may permit a larger volume of gas to be delivered than what is set in volume-control mode, and some ventilators will not register an accurate exhaled tidal volume. For this reason, pressure-control ventilation is preferable. The inspiratory pressure should be set at a level sufficient to attain rise of the chest and provide acceptable (if not normal) alveolar ventilation. In order to avoid barotrauma, keeping the inspiratory pressure less than 30 cm H_2O is advised, if possible. If volume-control ventilation is desired, then the clinician should either use a conversion table for the particular ventilator being used[21] to estimate the true tidal volume, or else periodically measure the exhaled tidal volume at the level of the endotracheal tube with a density-independent pneumotachograph.[22] Using pressure-control ventilation is easier.

The second issue is the FiO_2. Most ventilators have two gas inlets—one for 100% oxygen, and one for air (21% oxygen). The gas blender will mix the two to attain the FiO_2 selected on the ventilator. Administration of helium through the air inlet can result in a different FiO_2 actually delivered to the patient. In the case of pure helium going through the air inlet, the delivered FiO_2 may be less than what's selected (normally the air inlet has 21% oxygen, and with pure helium there's 0% oxygen). More commonly, a premixed Heliox tank is connected to the air inlet. If the Heliox is, say, 70% helium and 30% oxygen, and the FiO_2 on the vent is set at 30% oxygen, then the patient will end up receiving a higher FiO_2 than the selected 30% (due to mixture of the gases). This may reduce the efficacy of the Heliox, especially if the true FiO_2 exceeds 40%. It can also increase the volume of gas delivered to the patient and increase the airway pressures. To make this even more complicated, different ventilators use different mixing valves and blenders. It's important to know how the particular ventilators you're using work with Heliox.

There are two ways around the issue of the FiO_2. The first is to directly sample the inspired gas with a density-independent measuring device, which is cumbersome. The second is to connect a premixed tank of Heliox to the air inlet of the ventilator, and set the FiO_2 on the vent to 21%. This means that no supplemental oxygen is added to the Heliox mixture and that only the Heliox is delivered to the patient. The gas blender on the tank, or the mixture of the gas in the tank itself, can be used to control the "true" FiO_2—the vent may say the FiO_2 is 21%, but if the tank is full of 70:30 Heliox, then the patient is actually getting 30% oxygen. This is the easiest method, but it requires informing the nursing and respiratory staff that the FiO_2 is not actually 21% (despite what it says on the ventilator).

Ketamine

Ketamine is a dissociative agent that has marked sedative and analgesic properties, and it's most commonly used for procedural sedation. Unlike benzodiazepines, which act on inhibitory GABA receptors, ketamine blocks excitatory NMDA receptors in the central nervous system. NMDA receptors are also present in the lungs and appear to play a role in bronchoconstriction. Ketamine's anti-NMDA effect would therefore make it an attractive agent to use in conditions of severe bronchospasm like status asthmaticus. Experimental models have also suggested that ketamine has a salutary effect on bronchospasm through effects on norepinephrine reuptake and vagal inhibition.[23]

Ketamine is not without side effects. The most commonly reported is an increase in airway secretions. Psychiatric side effects have also been described, including disorientation and hallucinations. It should be noted that the psychiatric side effects are more common with higher doses of ketamine, especially when it is used for general anesthesia.[24] Benzodiazepines can ameliorate these side effects. Other adverse reactions to ketamine include laryngospasm, hypertension, and increased intracranial pressure.

Clinical trials report mixed results, with some demonstrating an improvement in airway pressures, gas exchange, and bronchospasm. Others have not been as supportive of using this agent in mechanically ventilated asthmatics. At this time, no large, randomized, prospective trials have been performed to support or discourage the use of ketamine in the setting of severe bronchospasm. As such, it should be considered a rescue agent to be used when conventional therapy (steroids, bronchodilators, appropriate ventilation settings, and adequate sedation) has proven ineffective.

The typical dosing for ketamine in status asthmaticus has not been clearly defined. Clinical trials have used an initial bolus anywhere from 0.1 mg/kg to 2.0 mg/kg, followed by infusions ranging from 0.15 mg/kg/hr to 2.5 mg/kg/hr for up to five days.[23] Because of the lack of clear evidence-based recommendations, it seems prudent to start with a lower bolus dose like 0.1 to 0.5 mg/kg, followed by an infusion starting at 0.15 to 0.25 mg/kg/hr. The infusion can be titrated upward until the desired clinical response of adequate sedation, improvement in gas exchange, and improvement in bronchospasm (as determined by chest auscultation and lower airway pressures) is attained. Furthermore, it makes sense to administer benzodiazepines when the ketamine is being weaned off to prevent emergence reactions.

Therapeutic Bronchoscopy

Therapeutic bronchoscopy is occasionally necessary to clear the airways of thick mucus plugs and bronchial casts. Occlusion of large conducting airways can definitely affect lung mechanics and gas exchange, and seems to limit the delivery of inhaled bronchodilators to smaller airways. One review of 93 cases of fatal asthma showed that airway obstruction by exudative secretions was a significant cause of death.[25] Early evaluation of the tracheobronchial tree with fiberoptic bronchoscopy should be considered in patients with severe bronchospasm, and mucus plugs should be aggressively lavaged.

Giving mucolytics like N-acetylcysteine through the bronchoscope may be helpful, but this can cause bronchospasm. Instrumentation of the airways themselves with the bronchoscope can also cause immediate or delayed bronchospasm. For "routine" cases of asthma, bronchoscopy is probably not warranted and may cause complications. For severe cases, however, the likelihood of significant mucus plugging or casting of the airways is higher and the benefits of bronchoalveolar lavage may outweigh the risk.

Wait It Out

One of the major challenges in the critical care of patients with severe bronchospasm is that they don't get better right away. It may take several days or longer for the steroids and bronchodilators to take effect and for the inflammation and bronchospasm to subside. In the meantime, it is important to stay focused on the following goals:

- Maintain adequate (but not perfect) oxygenation—an SpO_2 88-95% is fine. Hyperoxia isn't necessary or helpful.

- Reduce hyperinflation by giving the lungs plenty of time to exhale.

- Tolerate a respiratory acidosis, especially if "normalizing" the $PaCO_2$ and pH means injuring the lungs with high tidal volumes or dynamic hyperinflation. Prevention of ventilator-induced lung injury is far more important than a "good" ABG. Let the pH go down as low as 7.10 if necessary.

- Use therapies like Heliox, ketamine, and therapeutic bronchoscopy if necessary, but don't let them distract you from the goals listed above.

59

- Provide good holistic critical care. That includes nutritional support, DVT prophylaxis, and mobilization when appropriate.
- Be patient. It takes time to get better. Put the patient on the right course, monitor for changes, and let your plan work. In an age of instant gratification, this can be the hardest part!

Chapter Six

Prone Positioning and Neuromuscular Blockade

Two adjunctive strategies for treating severe ARDS that have been used for years are prone positioning and therapeutic neuromuscular blockade. These are often used in conjunction with each other, and the clinical rationale is improved ventilator-perfusion matching and alveolar recruitment. Until recently, neither treatment had shown an improvement in survival from severe respiratory failure (although there was proof of improved oxygenation).

In 2013, Guérin and colleagues published a multicenter randomized trial (PROSEVA) examining the effect of prone positioning for 16 hours, followed by 8 hours supine, in patients with ARDS.[26] They reported an overall reduction in mortality of 16.8%. In 2010, Papazian and colleagues published a multicenter, randomized, double-blind study (ACURASYS) that demonstrated a reduction in the hazard ratio for death from ARDS when a cisatracurium infusion was used for 48 hours early in the treatment of moderate-to-severe ARDS.[27] The publication of these two papers led to the inclusion of these therapies in professional guidelines and has prompted interest in these, and other, strategies for the treatment of ARDS.

Despite the enthusiasm that has greeted these findings, it's important to keep in mind that there are limitations with these and other studies, and that their findings should not result in wholesale application of prone positioning and neuromuscular blockade in every patient with ARDS. In this chapter, the pros and cons of each treatment will be discussed. If this seems like hedging, well, that's because it is. Both prone positioning and neuromuscular blockade have a place in the treatment of ARDS, and both have significant risks. Neither is a magic bullet, and neither is a substitute for lung-protective ventilation and good supportive critical care. By the time you're reading this, there may be new developments either supporting or refuting (or both!) these therapies. For now, the focus should be on identifying the patients who may benefit while minimizing the risks.

In Favor Of Prone Positioning

In ARDS, dorsal lung units tend to become more consolidated. Transpulmonary pressures are increased in dorsal alveoli and lower in ventral alveoli. At the same time, the gravitational effect on pulmonary blood flow leads to these units being relatively more perfused than the aerated ventral lung units. This has the effect of increasing the shunt fraction and worsening oxygenation. The rationale for prone positioning is that flipping the patient onto his abdomen will improve ventilation-perfusion matching and thereby improve gas exchange. At the same time, a more even distribution of aeration and transpulmonary pressure occurs.

There are other benefits as well. Prone positioning improves drainage of pulmonary secretions from the airways. Allowing the abdominal contents to be dependent (by padding the patient's chest and pelvis) reduces the pressure on the diaphragm and improves chest wall compliance. The weight of the heart, which is normally directed over the left lower lobe, is shifted centrally.

Previous studies of prone positioning were able to show improvement in pulmonary blood flow and oxygenation, but did not improve mortality.[28,29] This may have been due to using prone positioning in patients with less-severe ARDS, poorly-defined protocols, and a shorter duration of the time spent prone. The 2013 Guérin study, on the other hand, was well-defined and included patients with a PaO_2/FiO_2 ratio $\leq$ 150. These patients were sufficiently ill enough to where a treatment benefit might become evident. This study also mandated that the time spent prone (16 hours at a time) was long enough for any physiologic benefit to occur. Earlier studies had prone times of 6-8 hours.

The risks of prone positioning include dislodgement of life support equipment like endotracheal tubes and vascular catheters; pressure injury to the eyes, face, and extremities; and the need for heavy sedation and often neuromuscular blockade. Many of these complications can be reduced or avoided by using a clearly-defined protocol for turning and adequate staff training. While sedation and neuromuscular blockade have risks, limiting prone positioning to those patients who have moderate-to-severe ARDS (and stopping it once the patients begin to recover) should keep the number of days spent heavily sedated down.

Arguments Against Prone Positioning

The centers that participated in the PROSEVA trial have ample experience with prone positioning for ARDS. The importance of staff education and protocols for proning cannot be overstated. The risks to both the patient and to the staff are highest during the turning process. Intensive care units that wish to make this a part of how they care for ARDS should develop checklists and practice doing it so that it can happen seamlessly when actually done for critically ill patients.

63

The PROSEVA trial did show a mortality benefit, but it's important to note that it was the first trial of prone positioning in ARDS to do so after numerous other clinical trials had failed. This may have been due to improvement in the process and a refinement of the indications and duration of treatment. It could also easily reflect the fact that clinical statistics are not exact and that occasionally a trial can demonstrate a benefit when none actually exists. The PROSEVA trial was very similar to another clinical study of prone positioning published in 2009.[30] That study looked at a similar number of patients (466, vs. 342 in PROSEVA) and included patients with a PaO_2/FiO_2 ratio $\leq$ 200. It also used a similar duration of proning (20 hours at a time, vs. 16 hours in PROSEVA). There was the expected improvement in oxygenation, but no statistically significant difference in mortality. The fact that two very similar clinical trials reached very different conclusions suggests that a much larger tie-breaker trial is needed.

The final issue that clinicians should consider with PROSEVA is the overall reduction in mortality. There was a nearly 17% absolute risk reduction, which is **huge**. No other treatment in critical care medicine has been able to consistently reduce the risk of death that much. This may be a case of "if it looks too good to be true, it probably is."

In Favor of Therapeutic Neuromuscular Blockade

Much of the ventilator-induced lung injury seen in ARDS is due to high transpulmonary pressure in vulnerable alveoli and overdistension of relatively healthy lung units during mechanical ventilation. Therapeutic neuromuscular blockade, along with heavy sedation, aims to improve respiratory system compliance and patient-ventilator dyssynchrony. Inflammatory biomarkers in both the blood and in bronchoalveolar fluid are also reduced when neuromuscular blockade is used.[31] These effects putatively lower the risk of ventilator-induced lung injury and improve survival from ARDS.

The ACURASYS trial used a bolus of cisatracurium, followed by a continuous infusion, for 48 hours early in the treatment of moderate-to-severe ARDS ($PaO_2/FiO_2 \leq 150$). This led to an improvement in the hazard ratio of death at 90 days, along with a reduction in the incidence of pneumothorax (4% vs. 11.7%). The benefit was most pronounced in patients with a PaO_2/FiO_2 ratio ≤ 120, suggesting that neuromuscular blockade is most effective in the sickest patients. Other, smaller clinical trials have also suggested that a cisatracurium infusion may be beneficial.[31,32] Importantly, these trials did not show a higher risk of prolonged myopathy or ICU-acquired weakness when compared with the control groups.

Arguments Against Neuromuscular Blockade

The ACURASYS trial claimed a reduction in the 90-day hazard ratio of death, but the overall reduction in mortality was not statistically significant. In other words, patients who received cisatracurium lived longer than the control arm, but a similar number were dead by the 90-day mark. A reduction in the hazard ratio may be a meaningful outcome in a trial looking at a new treatment for, say, lung cancer—the five-year mortality may not be different, but the new drug may prolong life for another year or two. Most people would consider that successful. Most people would probably not consider an additional week or two of life in the ICU, intubated and attached to machines, to be a successful result.

There are also concerns regarding the external validity of the study. The rate of pneumothorax in the control group was nearly 12%, which seems higher than what's seen in clinical practice. This leads to questions regarding the ventilator strategy used, and it turns out that the prescribed tidal volume in this trial was 6-8 mL/kg PBW. This is a higher tidal volume than what's recommended for moderate-to-severe ARDS. Another trial using a lower tidal volume strategy would seem to be needed.

Nearly 22% of the control group in the ACURASYS trial received open-label cisatracurium. This makes interpretation of the results difficult, as the study wasn't completely blinded. Patients with more pronounced dyssynchrony with the ventilator would be the ones expected to receive open-label neuromuscular blockade, and these would also be the ones in the control group. In an effort to preserve blinding, all patients in the study had to be sedated to the point of complete unresponsiveness prior to receiving either the cisatracurium infusion or placebo. Heavy sedation is also known to be associated with higher risks. These issues should not be discounted.

Lastly, much of the improvement in critical care medicine over the last 15-20 years has been with the realization that "less is more." Heavy sedation and routine neuromuscular blockade have given way to daily awakening trials and analgesia-first sedation strategies. Mobilization of critically ill patients is becoming more accepted, as is recognition and prevention of delirium. Implementation of the ACURASYS method could be a step backwards.

Putting It Together

The point of the preceding arguments was not to convince you that all patients with ARDS should be proned and paralyzed, and it wasn't intended to say that proning and neuromuscular blockade are worthless. The truth is that both may have a role in moderate-to-severe ARDS ($PaO_2/FiO_2 \leq 150$), and they should be considered on a case-by-case basis. The patients most likely to benefit from prone positioning are those with significant dorsal consolidation as seen on CT imaging. Patients with more diffuse infiltrates may not see as much of a response to changes in respiratory mechanics and pulmonary blood flow. Additionally, the nursing care of other issues (long bone fractures, recent chest or abdominal surgery, brain injury, etc.) may be adversely affected with proning. Proper training and drilling of ICU staff, along with the use of a proning checklist, should minimize the risk of turning to both patients and caregivers.

The patients most likely to benefit from therapeutic neuromuscular blockade include those with extremely poor respiratory compliance; those with significant dyssynchrony with the ventilator despite the best efforts of the clinician; and those with coexisting issues like abdominal compartment syndrome or intracranial hypertension where an improvement in thoracic compliance could lead to an overall improvement in hemodynamics and end-organ perfusion. Neuromuscular blockade should be questioned in patients receiving high-dose corticosteroids due to the higher risk of ICU-acquired weakness syndrome.

For this reason as well, cisatracurium (a benzylisoquinolone that is metabolized in the plasma by Hofmann degradation) is preferred over aminosteroidal neuromuscular blockers like vecuronium or pancuronium—these agents have a higher risk of ICU-acquired weakness when concomitantly administered with steroids. They (the aminosteroidal drugs) also depend on hepatic and renal metabolism and their effects may be prolonged with hepatic or renal dysfunction, which are quite common in the ICU. Peripheral nerve stimulation should be used to monitor the depth of neuromuscular blockade, and a daily sedation/paralytic holiday should be considered.

Prone Positioning Checklist

Indications For Prone Positioning
Hypoxemic respiratory failure with the following features:
- PaO_2/FiO_2 ratio ≤ 150
- Diffuse bilateral lung infiltrates
- Dorsal consolidation on CT (if available)

Minimum Necessary Personnel
- 2 respiratory therapists (or other qualified personnel) to control the airway and ventilator
- 4 turners (may be nurse, physician, patient care tech, respiratory therapist, or student)
- 1 supervisor, who should not be involved in the proning process itself

Turning Process

PREPARE
- Apply lubricant to eyes and tape eyelids closed
- Remove any jewelry from the patient's head or neck
- Remove any bite blocks
- Bolus necessary analgesia/sedation/neuromuscular blocker
- Confirm SpO_2 and $ETCO_2$ monitors are in place and functional

POSITION
- Two turners on either side of the patient (four total)
- Two respiratory therapists at the head of the patient
  - One to manage the head, airway, and face pillow
  - One to manage ventilator tubing and provide backup
- Supervisor at the foot of the bed

PAD (if going from SUPINE to PRONE)
- Foam face pillow, making sure the endotracheal tube is not kinked (it may be necessary to cut out some of the foam padding)
- Two pillows each on the chest, lower pelvis, and shins
- Place a sheet over the patient (head to toe) and wrap snugly, bundling the pillows to the patient

DISCONNECT
- Central lines (after necessary boluses)
- Arterial lines
- Hemodialysis lines
- Cardiac monitor leads
- The endotracheal tube from the ventilator
    o Attach a self-inflating bag connected to oxygen
    o Adjust the PEEP valve on the bag to the appropriate level, based on the patient's oxygenation
    o Put the ventilator on standby

TURN
Supervisor should read each step aloud, with verbal confirmation by the team members

o Supervisor confirms that the airway and ventilator tubing are under control by the respiratory therapists

o Supervisor confirms that all lines and leads have been disconnected (SpO$_2$ and ETCO$_2$ monitors may be left in place, unless they interfere with the turning process)

o On the supervisor's count, the team will turn the patient onto his **left/right** (specify which) side, keeping the pillows tight against the body using the sheet

o Supervisor confirms that nothing needs to be repositioned

o On the supervisor's count, the team will turn the patient to the **PRONE** or **SUPINE** position, ensuring that the pillows and face pad are kept in the proper position

o Respiratory therapists confirm to the supervisor that the endotracheal tube is at the proper depth and that the tube is not obstructed, with an appropriate $ETCO_2$ waveform

o If **PRONE**, Turners confirm to the supervisor that the patient is appropriately padded and that arms and legs are positioned comfortably

o If **SUPINE**, Turners remove padding

o Reattach cardiac monitor leads, arterial line, and restart infusions

Prone position should be maintained for 16 hours, followed by 8 hours in the supine position. Eye and mouth care is essential. Tube feeding in the prone position is permissible if the tube is post-pyloric; otherwise, hold tube feeding while prone and increase the rate of feeding while supine.

Chapter Seven

Inhaled Pulmonary Vasodilators

Positive airway pressure has a beneficial effect on left ventricular function by reducing both preload and afterload (the transmural pressure across the left ventricle). At the same time, however, positive airway pressure can worsen right ventricular function—the normally low-pressure pulmonary vascular circuit now is subjected to significant pressure from the ventilator. Hypoxic pulmonary vasoconstriction also increases the workload on the right ventricle. Most of the time, this doesn't affect hemodynamics too much, and fluid loading is sufficient to maintain right ventricular output. In some patients, though, pulmonary hypertension and right ventricular dysfunction can have a notably adverse effect on both cardiac and pulmonary function.

Right ventricular (RV) dysfunction and even overt RV failure can be seen with severe ARDS. It is also seen with massive or submassive pulmonary embolism, right ventricular infarction, and in patients with preexisting pulmonary hypertension (chronic obstructive pulmonary disease, obstructive sleep apnea, connective tissue diseases, primary pulmonary hypertension, etc.). RV failure can be particularly difficult to treat—the right ventricle is normally a thin-walled structure that operates best in conditions of low vascular pressure and resistance. A sudden increase in pulmonary vascular resistance is hard for the RV to deal with—it just doesn't have the muscle mass of the left ventricle. Inotropes like milrinone and dobutamine can be used to "whip the heart," but an increase in cardiac output is often neutralized by a corresponding rise in myocardial oxygen consumption. In this situation, a selective pulmonary arterial vasodilator may prove to be helpful.

The most commonly used pulmonary arterial dilator in critical care medicine is inhaled nitric oxide (iNO). iNO can be delivered by mask or through the endotracheal tube and has a rapid vasodilatory effect on pulmonary arterioles and capillaries. One particular advantage of iNO is that it will only cause vasodilation in the alveolar-capillary beds that it reaches. This has the effect of improving ventilation-perfusion matching in patients with severe hypoxemia. Inhaled prostacyclin can also be used and has the same physiologic effect. Intravenous pulmonary vasodilators like prostacyclin and alprostadil can be used, but tend to have a much more potent effect on hemodynamic function and often cause hypotension.

There have not been many clinical trials of inhaled prostacyclin, and the evidence base is limited. iNO has been studied much more extensively, and so further discussion will center on the use of iNO. This does not mean that inhaled prostacyclin is not effective, and it may work just as well as iNO in similar clinical settings. It is important to note that neither iNO nor inhaled prostacyclin are FDA-approved for use in adults with ARDS or right ventricular failure, and any use is off-label.

The allure of inhaled pulmonary vasodilators is that they cause selective vasodilation only in the lung units that they can reach; they have a rapid onset and offset; that they have minimal adverse hemodynamic effects; and that there are no downstream metabolites. For years, this was thought to be the case. iNO was believed to be inactivated immediately by reacting with hemoglobin in the pulmonary capillaries. Recent research has shown that this is not the case. iNO reacts with hemoglobin and leads to formation of nitrite and S-nitrosohemoglobin. Nitrite can be recycled in downstream tissues to nitric oxide, which can cause systemic capillary vasodilation. S-nitrosohemoglobin also induces nitric oxide production, particularly in the setting of tissue hypoxia. This couples vasodilation and deoxygenation, which may lead to mitochondrial dysfunction. This has been demonstrated in clinical trials, where use of iNO is associated with a higher rate of renal failure.[33] Presumably, the toxic effects of these metabolites are not limited to the kidneys, which means that the metabolites of iNO could contribute to multisystem organ dysfunction.

iNO and ARDS

In patients with ARDS, iNO may improve oxygenation via selective pulmonary vasodilatation. No studies have shown a survival benefit with this therapy, however, and a recent meta-analysis[34] of nine clinical trials concluded that, "Nitric oxide does not reduce mortality in adults or children with acute respiratory distress syndrome, regardless of the degree of hypoxemia." The reason for the lack of benefit seems to be in line with other therapies that have been shown to improve oxygenation but not survival—very few patients with ARDS die of refractory hypoxemia. The majority die of multisystem organ failure, and the potentially toxic metabolites of iNO may potentiate this. Therefore, iNO should only be used in ARDS as a true rescue therapy. It may be helpful in patients with a PaO_2/FiO_2 ratio less than 55 despite optimal care and who are not candidates for other rescue therapies that have been proven to be beneficial (prone positioning, veno-venous ECMO).

iNO and Right Ventricular Failure

Acute right ventricular failure is primarily treated with fluid loading and inotropic support. Dobutamine and milrinone are inotropes that increase right ventricular contractility. Milrinone, a phosphodiesterase-III inhibitor, also has vasodilatory properties on the pulmonary circulation. Levosimendan is another calcium-sensitizing inodilator, but it is not commercially available in the United States.

RV failure is often associated with moderate-to-severe hypoxemia and pulmonary dysfunction. Conventional ventilator strategies that use high levels of PEEP or increase the mean airway pressure (like APRV) can worsen right ventricular function and increase pulmonary vascular pressures. Inhaled nitric oxide or prostacyclin can be used to lower the pulmonary vascular resistance, thereby improving right ventricular function and improving gas exchange.

When initiating inhaled pulmonary vasodilators for right ventricular failure, a pulmonary artery catheter is strongly encouraged. Echocardiography can also be used to evaluate contractility and to measure pulmonary artery pressure, but it isn't available continuously and is not ideal for titrating medications. The pulmonary artery catheter can continuously measure pulmonary artery pressure, cardiac output, and SvO_2. It can also be used to calculate the pulmonary vascular resistance. This is very useful for differentiating between conditions that cause pulmonary arterial hypertension and those associated with pulmonary venous hypertension. Selective pulmonary vasodilators tend to be more effective for the former.

Pulmonary vascular resistance (PVR) can be calculated by measuring the mean pulmonary artery pressure and the pulmonary artery occlusion pressure at end-expiration. The difference between the two measurements is then divided by the cardiac output (in L/min).

$$PVR = [mean\ PAP - PAOP] / [CO]$$

A patient with a normal mean pulmonary artery pressure (20 mm Hg), pulmonary artery occlusion pressure (10 mm Hg), and cardiac output (5 L/min) would have a pulmonary vascular resistance of 2 mm Hg-min/L, or Wood units. Normal PVR is 2-3 Wood units.* Conditions that elevate both the mean PAP and the PAOP (most commonly left ventricular dysfunction, but also mitral and aortic valvular disease) are characterized by pulmonary hypertension and a normal PVR. This is often referred to as pulmonary venous hypertension. The high pressure in the left atrium leads to high right-sided pressures in order to keep the blood flowing. Caution should be used with any kind of pulmonary vasodilator—lowering the mean PAP, while the PAOP remains elevated, often leads to pulmonary edema.

Consider a patient who has severe systolic CHF. He has a mean PAP of 40 mm Hg and a PAOP of 30 mm Hg. The PAOP (a.k.a. the wedge pressure) represents left atrial pressure. Left atrial pressure equals left ventricular pressure at the end of diastole, when blood stops flowing from the atrium to the ventricle. The left ventricular end-diastolic pressure is elevated due to severe CHF. The only way that blood can flow from the right ventricle through the pulmonary vasculature and into the left ventricle is if the pulmonary artery pressure is higher than the left ventricular pressure. Now, this patient is started on iNO. The mean PAP falls, as predicted. iNO is a selective pulmonary vasodilator, which means that it will not reduce the left ventricular afterload. The left atrial pressure remains the same. If the mean PAP is now 28, and the left atrial pressure is 30, you can see where this is going. Blood flow will reverse, leading to pulmonary edema and hypotension.

Pulmonary arterial hypertension, on the other hand, is characterized by an imbalance between the mean PAP and the PAOP. Thromboembolic disease, connective tissue disease, and chronic hypoxemia are common causes. A patient with a mean PAP of 45 mm Hg, PAOP of 15 mm Hg, and a cardiac output of 6

---

* PVR is often expressed in dyne-sec-cm^{-5}. This is obtained by multiplying the number of Wood units by 79.9. I'm not sure why this is. I find it easier to use Wood units.

L/min has PVR of 5 Wood units, suggesting pulmonary arterial hypertension. Right ventricular dysfunction with a PVR $\geq$ 4 Wood units may improve with a pulmonary vasodilator.

It is important to remember that inhaled nitric oxide or prostacyclin is an adjunctive therapy, and not a treatment in itself. The underlying condition leading to right ventricular failure should be treated aggressively. Pulmonary embolism should be treated with anticoagulation and thrombolysis. Acute chest syndrome in patients with sickle cell disease should be treated with antibiotics and exchange transfusion. Acute myocardial infarction should be treated with reperfusion therapy. Attention to volume status is crucial—while hypovolemia will certainly lead to hypotension, volume overload will cause bowing of the interventricular septum and compromise left ventricular filling. Euvolemia, guided by echocardiography and/or pulmonary artery catheter monitoring, should be achieved by diuresis or renal replacement therapy.

Administration of iNO and Inhaled Prostacyclin

iNO is available with a commercial delivery system that has a long track record of reliability and safety. Using an unapproved, self-made delivery system has the risk of unreliable dosing of iNO and potentially toxic exposure of the patient and staff to nitrogen dioxide. Use the commercial system!

Inhaled prostacyclin can be reconstituted in saline and delivered by a jet nebulizer system modified for use with mechanical ventilation. This requires an aerosol delivery device that can be coordinated with the ventilator's inspiratory cycle, which has been described in the literature.[35]

Initial Dosing of iNO

iNO should be started at 20 parts per million (ppm). A successful response is a reduction in the mean pulmonary artery pressure by at least 10%, and usually an improvement in the PaO_2 by at least 20 mm Hg. If the patient does not respond within 5-10 minutes, then a higher concentration (40 ppm, or even 80 ppm) can be tried. Most patients who are going to respond will do so at 20 ppm. iNO should be stopped in those patients who do not have an initial response to therapy.

In patients who respond, the dose of iNO should be lowered in 5-10 ppm increments every 15-30 minutes, to a floor of 5 ppm. An increase in the mean PAP by $\geq$ 5 mm Hg, or a fall in the SpO_2 by $\geq$ 5%, should be treated by increasing the dose of iNO back to the level where it was effective.

iNO Initial Dosing Algorithm

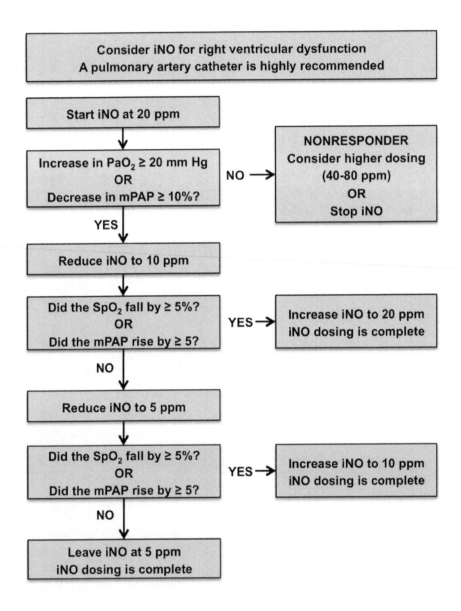

Weaning iNO

Once the patient has begun showing signs of recovery (improvement in gas exchange, less need for inotropes), iNO can be reduced or stopped altogether. This should be done slowly, as abrupt discontinuation of the drug can lead to rebound hypoxemia and pulmonary hypertension.

When the patient is tolerating an iNO dose of 5 ppm, the drug can be weaned off. The iNO dose should be lowered by 1 ppm every 30 minutes. If the mean PAP increases by $\geq$ 5 mm Hg, or the SpO_2 falls by $\geq$ 5%, the iNO should be returned to 5 ppm and further attempts at weaning should be postponed for at least 12 hours. Once the iNO is at 2 ppm, a single dose of sildenafil 20 mg can be given (if it's not already being administered). This may help prevent rebound pulmonary hypertension as the drug is weaned off. After administration of the sildenafil, continue to reduce the iNO by 1 ppm every 30 minutes until it's off.

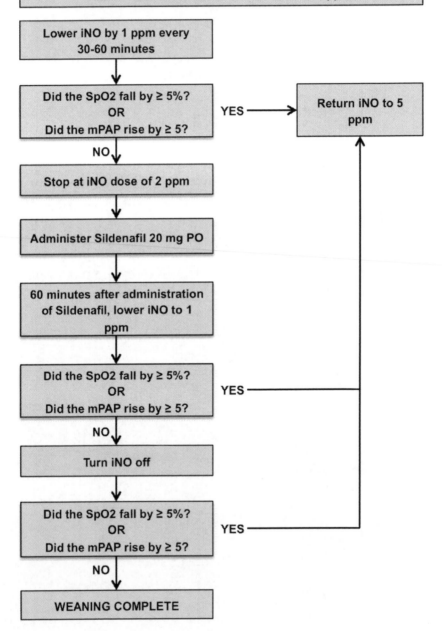

Begin weaning iNO once the patient's hemodynamics and respiratory status have stabilized at an iNO dose of 5 ppm

Lower iNO by 1 ppm every 30-60 minutes

Did the SpO2 fall by ≥ 5%?
OR
Did the mPAP rise by ≥ 5?

YES → Return iNO to 5 ppm

NO

Stop at iNO dose of 2 ppm

Administer Sildenafil 20 mg PO

60 minutes after administration of Sildenafil, lower iNO to 1 ppm

Did the SpO2 fall by ≥ 5%?
OR
Did the mPAP rise by ≥ 5?

YES

NO

Turn iNO off

Did the SpO2 fall by ≥ 5%?
OR
Did the mPAP rise by ≥ 5?

YES

NO

WEANING COMPLETE

Chapter Eight

Veno-Venous ECMO

There are times when a patient's lung disease is so severe that adequate gas exchange is either impossible, or can only be accomplished with prohibitively high airway pressures and tidal volumes. When this is the case, veno-venous extracorporeal membrane oxygenation (VV ECMO) should be considered as a rescue therapy. This chapter is simply an overview of the use of extracorporeal support and is designed to familiarize the reader with the rationale for its use. Those desiring to treat patients with ECMO are strongly encouraged to attend a training program sponsored by the Extracorporeal Life Support Organization (ELSO).

VV vs. VA

Veno-venous ECMO is considerably different from veno-arterial ECMO (VA ECMO). VA ECMO is similar to heart-lung bypass. Blood is drained from the venous side using a cannula placed in the femoral vein. The blood is pumped through an oxygenator, and the fully oxygenated blood is returned to the patient via a cannula placed in the femoral or subclavian artery (Figure 1). In neonates, the carotid artery is often used; in adults, however, the carotid artery is avoided due to the risk of stroke. With VA ECMO, the extracorporeal circuit can support both the pulmonary and the cardiac systems. The flow through the pump can make up for even the most severe heart failure. In fact, the primary indication for VA ECMO in adults is refractory cardiogenic shock.

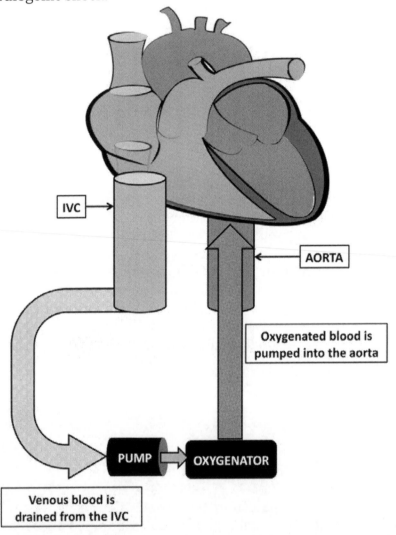

The VA ECMO circuit provides both respiratory and cardiac support by pumping oxygenated blood directly into the aorta. The pump flow is sufficient to replace the entire cardiac output, if necessary.

VV ECMO, on the other hand, provides no cardiac support. Blood is drained from the inferior vena cava through a cannula placed in the femoral vein. After being pumped through an oxygenator, the blood is returned to the right atrium through a cannula placed in the internal jugular vein.

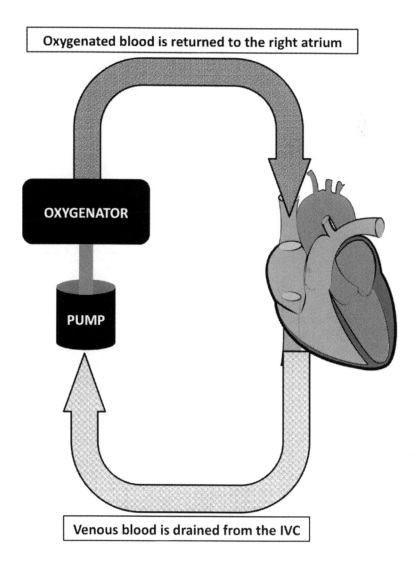

Dual-lumen cannulas are also available, and function similarly to dual-lumen hemodialysis catheters (albeit much larger, to accommodate a flow of 4-7 L/min). The dual-lumen cannula is placed via the right internal jugular vein. It passes through the superior vena cava and into the inferior vena cava. The siphon, or drainage, ports are at the tip of the cannula in the IVC. Using transesophageal echocardiography, the cannula is manipulated so that the return port is directed over the tricuspid valve. This helps reduce the risk of recirculation.

How VV ECMO Provides Respiratory Support

The best way to visualize VV ECMO is to consider the entire circuit as an extension of the right atrium. Normally, venous blood returning to the right atrium has an SvO_2 of 70-80%. In a markedly hypoxemic patient, the SvO_2 is much lower—50-60% is the norm. The venous blood goes through the pulmonary vascular system, where oxygen is picked up and CO_2 is unloaded (and ventilated off). Obviously, if a patient has severe ARDS, then the degree to which this gas exchange can occur is quite limited. Blood with an SvO_2 of 50% may only rise to an SaO_2 of 80%, even while the patient is breathing 100% oxygen and receiving high levels of PEEP.

When VV ECMO is initiated, some (but not all) of the venous blood is siphoned into the circuit. A pump drives a blood flow of 4-7 L/min through a membrane oxygenator. As the blood passes through the oxygenator, the hemoglobin becomes fully saturated and the PaO_2 may rise as high as 400-500 mm Hg. When this blood, with an SaO_2 of 100%, is returned to the right atrium, it mixes with the remaining venous blood and then proceeds through the pulmonary circulation. If half of the venous blood has an SvO_2 of 60% and the other half has an SvO_2 of 100% (thanks to the ECMO circuit), the total venous return going through the pulmonary circulation has an SvO_2 of roughly 80%. With higher pump flows, a greater percentage of the venous return is oxygenated using the ECMO circuit, leading to a higher overall SvO_2. In most patients, the ECMO flow can be increased to the point where the total SvO_2 is 85-90%.

Here's where VV ECMO becomes really cool. It's also where you have to remember the principles of oxygen delivery [see the earlier chapter in this book]. With a high enough cardiac output and hemoglobin, oxygen delivery to the tissues can be maintained even with mild-to-moderate hypoxemia. In other words, an SaO_2 of 80-85% is perfectly fine so long as cardiac output is sufficient and there is enough hemoglobin to carry the bound oxygen.

If an SaO_2 of 80-85% is enough to get the job done (with adequate cardiac output and hemoglobin), and if the SvO_2 can be kept at 80-85% with VV ECMO, then **there is no need for pulmonary gas exchange whatsoever.** This is a very important point, and is the cornerstone to understanding why VV ECMO can be an effective rescue therapy for severe ARDS. If the venous blood has an SvO_2 of 85% and it flows through lungs that contribute absolutely nothing, then the blood reaching the left atrium will have an SaO_2 of 85%. Since we've already established that an SaO_2 of 85% is sufficient if there's adequate cardiac output and hemoglobin, then there is no need to "beat up the lungs" with high PEEP, high ventilator rates, or any of the other usual things that are done for severe respiratory failure. Instead, the ventilator can be put on what are generally considered "rest settings."

Ventilator Rest Settings on VV ECMO[*]

- Pressure Control Ventilation
- Rate 10 breaths/minute
- I-time 1.0-2.0 seconds, adjusted for comfort
- P_{INSP} 25 cm H_2O
- PEEP 10 cm H_2O
- FiO_2 30%

Gas exchange in the ECMO circuit is a function of blood flow through the oxygenator and the gas flow of oxygen across the oxygenator's membrane. The oxygen that is flowing across the membrane is known as the sweep gas because it "sweeps off" CO_2 from the blood in the membrane. CO_2 has a much higher solubility than oxygen, and so it can be rapidly eliminated by increasing the sweep gas flow. Oxygenation can be increased by raising the rate of blood flow through the membrane oxygenator. Put simply, circuit flow controls oxygenation, while the flow of sweep gas controls ventilation. Sweep gas is usually 2-6 L/min. The FiO_2 of the sweep gas is initially set at 1.0 in order to attain the best oxygenation of the blood in the circuit.

---

[*] Always remember that the whole point of VV ECMO for respiratory failure is to let the lungs rest and recover. If they look whited-out on the CXR and the tidal volume on these settings is < 100 mL, so be it! Resist the temptation to use the vent for gas exchange. Let the ECMO circuit do the work.

> **Initial VV ECMO Settings**
>
> - Circuit blood flow of 50-60 mL/kg
> - Adjust circuit flow to keep patient SaO_2 80-85%
> - FiO_2 on sweep gas of 100%
> - Set the sweep gas flow about the same as the circuit flow
> - Adjust sweep gas flow to keep $PaCO_2$ 35-45

Most of the time, some ventilator support is necessary. This isn't to provide additional gas exchange support, but instead to improve patient comfort and to prevent complications. If a patient is put on VV ECMO and then extubated, the lack of any positive pressure on the lungs will lead to near-complete alveolar collapse and consolidation. This can cause significant tachypnea and respiratory distress. Alveolar consolidation also prevents the normal clearance of secretions from the pulmonary tree, which can lead to pneumonia or lung abscess.

That said, recent experience with VV ECMO has shown that as patients recover, they can spend more and more time off the ventilator. This is important because it means that physical therapy and mobilization can begin early on, even while on VV ECMO. This is much easier with the dual-lumen cannula placed through the internal jugular vein. Early tracheostomy should be done as soon as it's feasible in order to lessen sedation and begin mobilization. There is nothing like seeing a patient with severe ARDS walk down the hallway, with the ECMO circuit being pushed behind him.

Weaning VV ECMO

As the patient begins to recover, the FiO_2 of the sweep gas can be lowered. Circuit flow, once established, should not be lowered—lower blood flow increases the risk of thrombosis in the circuit. Keep in mind that VV ECMO is just like a really big right atrium. As the FiO_2 on the sweep gas is reduced, the blood flowing through the oxygenator will pick up less oxygen. That means that the proportion of gas exchange that has to occur through the patient's lungs is increasing. Once the FiO_2 on the sweep gas is 0.21, the ECMO circuit is contributing nothing at all to the patient's oxygenation—it's all being done with low-level ventilator support. Blood is simply flowing through the big right atrium but there's no assistance with oxygenation. If the patient's condition is acceptable, it's time to come off ECMO.

Patient Selection

This is often the most difficult part of using VV ECMO for severe acute respiratory failure. For many years, ECMO was used predominantly for neonates with infant respiratory distress syndrome, meconium aspiration, and congenital diaphragmatic hernia. In recent years, however, ECMO has become more popular for older children and adults. The H1N1 influenza pandemic of 2009 accelerated the interest in ECMO, particularly VV ECMO, as a rescue therapy. The CESAR trial, published in *The Lancet* in 2009, demonstrated a survival benefit for patients with severe influenza-related ARDS transferred to ECMO centers.[36] Only 75% of those randomized to the ECMO arm actually received ECMO, which is an interesting finding. It may be that the true benefit was treating patients in high-volume centers with the appropriate expertise and ability to provide rescue therapies, including ECMO, rather than the provision of ECMO itself.

Indications for VV-ECMO

- Hypoxic respiratory failure with a predicted mortality risk $\geq 50\%$
  a. $PaO_2/FiO_2 < 150$ on $FiO_2 > 90\%$ despite optimal care for 6 hours or more
  b. Murray Score[*] ≥ 3 despite optimal care for 6 hours or more
- Hypercapnic respiratory failure refractory to treatment with pH < 7.15
- Acute onset of a potentially reversible cause of respiratory failure
- Age ≤ 65
- Immediate respiratory collapse that is unresponsive to optimal care (obstructed airway, etc.)

Contraindications to VV-ECMO[†]

- Mechanical ventilation at high settings (e.g. $FiO_2 \geq 90\%$, $P_{PLAT} > 30$, PEEP ≥ 15) for 7 days or longer
- Contraindication to anticoagulation
- Absolute neutrophil count $< 500/mm^3$
- Major CNS damage or other nonreversible comorbidity
- Age > 65
- Progression of chronic respiratory disease to the point of respiratory failure

---

[*] http://cesar.lshtm.ac.uk/murrayscorecalculator.htm

[†] Contraindications are relative, not absolute; however, the presence of these conditions is associated with a higher risk of treatment failure.

Prior to initiation of VV-ECMO, the following steps should be taken to improve the patient's condition. These are listed in order of preference, although not all are required prior to cannulation for ECMO.

1. Lung protective ventilation using a tidal volume of 4-6 mL/kg predicted body weight, with PEEP according to the ARDSNet study protocol
2. Airway pressure release ventilation, with a P_{HIGH} up to 35 cm H_2O
3. Prone positioning for 16 hours, followed by supine positioning for 8 hours
4. Diuresis or CRRT to within 105% of dry weight, if hemodynamics permit
5. Bronchoscopy with therapeutic aspiration of the tracheobronchial tree

If the patient has not improved with the aforementioned therapy, VV ECMO team should be considered. Additional rescue maneuvers that can be tried include:

6. Inhaled nitric oxide
7. High frequency oscillatory ventilation

The Extracorporeal Life Support Organization (ELSO) provides extensive expert guidelines for patient selection and referral at its website: www.elso.org.

Ventilator Management on Veno-Arterial ECMO

The bulk of this chapter is concerned with VV ECMO as a rescue therapy for severe respiratory failure. The ventilator management in VV ECMO is quite easy—let the circuit do the heavy work, and use the ventilator to simply keep the lungs open without injuring them. It is quite common for the tidal volume to be less than 100 mL while on the rest settings described earlier, and that's fine—after all, the whole point of VV ECMO is to let the patient's lungs rest and recover.

With VA ECMO, on the other hand, it's important to keep in mind that while the ECMO circuit provides oxygenated blood into the aorta, the blood in the aortic root is more dependent on the patient's native cardiopulmonary function. That means that the blood flowing from the pulmonary circulation into the left atrium and ventricle is delivered preferentially into the coronary ostia and the aortic arch. In other words, oxygen delivery to the coronary arteries still depends on mechanical ventilatory support. The rest of the body, particularly the lower thorax and abdomen, gets its oxygen delivery from the ECMO circuit.

The exact degree to which different areas of the body are perfused depends on how strong the heart is. Consider a patient with zero native cardiac function. All of his arterial flow, including the coronary ostia, depends on the ECMO circuit flow. As he begins to recover cardiac function, the native heart will begin pumping blood into the aortic arch. As the heart grows stronger, it will perfuse more and more blood to the coronary arteries and the vessels coming off the aortic arch. This can lead to a situation where the lower half of the body is well-oxygenated by the ECMO circuit, while the upper body (including the brain) is relatively hypoxic. The management of the "blue nose syndrome" is beyond the scope of this chapter.

Therefore, simply putting a patient receiving VA ECMO on rest settings like you would do with VV ECMO risks myocardial hypoxia. A higher FiO_2 and PEEP may be necessary. Unlike with VV ECMO, ventilator settings should be adjusted to attain adequate gas exchange. The most accurate site for arterial blood gas monitoring depends on where the arterial ECMO cannula is located. In most cases, the cannula is placed in a femoral artery and into the descending aorta. After the coronary ostia, the next branch off the aortic arch is the right brachiocephalic artery. A blood gas specimen from a right radial arterial line will give the most accurate measure of the native heart's oxygen delivery. In the cases of central subclavian artery cannulation, there is much less discrepancy in regional oxygen delivery. The arterial line is generally placed in the radial artery on the opposite side from the subclavian artery cannula.

Chapter Nine

2 A.M.

Your mother was right—nothing good happens after 2 A.M. Especially in the ICU. If you get called to the bedside of a critically ill patient in the middle of the night, it is almost never going to be for good news.

This chapter is designed as a step-by-step approach to the mechanically ventilated patient who is either not getting better or deteriorating despite your best efforts. It begins with the things you should check when a patient has a sudden change in condition. Some of this is also discussed in *The Ventilator Book*, but it doesn't hurt to read it again. There is also a stepwise algorithm for escalating ventilator support for severe ARDS, as well as a guide to initial vent settings for acute lung injury and obstructive lung disease. Despite the title of this chapter, this information is useful any time of day.

First Things

Whenever a critically ill patient takes a turn for the worse, the initial assessment should go back to the ABCs. This is drilled repeatedly in Advanced Cardiac Life Support and Advanced Trauma Life Support courses, and for good reason. For a mechanically ventilated patient, think **Tube, Sounds, Sats**. Make sure the endotracheal tube is in place and is

93

patent—capnography is very helpful in this regard. Auscultate the chest to make sure there is bilateral air entry, and listen for wheezing or rales that might point you toward the reason for the patient's deterioration. Ensure that the patient is adequately oxygenated—hypoxemia can be due to a mechanical problem, a pulmonary issue, a cardiovascular issue, or a combination of any of these.

Another useful mnemonic for evaluating the crashing ventilated patient is **DOPES**[*]:

- **D**isplacement of the endotracheal tube—assess with capnography to make sure the tube is still in the trachea. Mainstem intubation can also make a ventilated patient get worse. The tube usually migrates down the right mainstem bronchus, so if breath sounds are not equal pull the tube back a few centimeters and reassess.

- **O**bstruction of the endotracheal tube—again, capnography can be helpful. A suction catheter that doesn't easily pass is another clue. Make sure the tube isn't kinked. Tube obstructions from secretions can sometimes be cleared with a bronchoscope or a CAM Rescue Cath™. If there's any doubt, take a look with a laryngoscope and reintubate the patient with a fresh tube.

- **P**neumothorax—chest X-ray is usually helpful but may not be immediately available. Bedside ultrasound can show a lack of pleural sliding. If there's concern for a tension pneumothorax (hypotension, hypoxemia, and absent breath sounds), emergent decompression should be strongly considered.

- **E**quipment malfunction—the best way to exclude this as a cause is to disconnect the patient from the ventilator, attach a self-inflating bag, and manually ventilate while further assessments are performed.

---

[*] http://wikem.org/wiki/deterioration_after_intubation

- **S**tacked breaths—this almost always happens in severe obstructive lung disease. Auto-PEEP can progress to the point where it causes hypotension or even pulselessness. A clue is when the patient is very difficult to manually ventilate and breath sounds are markedly diminished bilaterally. The treatment is disconnection of the vent or bag—if there's a rush of air out of the endotracheal tube, followed by hemodynamic improvement, then auto-PEEP is the culprit. Reconnect the patient to the ventilator with a lower respiratory rate and ensure that there's enough time for exhalation.

Initial Ventilator Setup

These are general guidelines for initial ventilator settings, divided between acute lung injury (sepsis, trauma, ARDS, pulmonary edema, etc.) and obstructive lung disease (asthma, COPD). The specific ventilator management of these patients must be individualized, and the general principles are described in more detail elsewhere. The purpose of these guidelines is to provide a quick reference that is applicable to the majority of patients placed on the ventilator in the ICU or the Emergency Department.

Acute Lung Injury Ventilator Setup
[ARDS, Sepsis, Trauma, Pneumonitis, Pulmonary Edema]

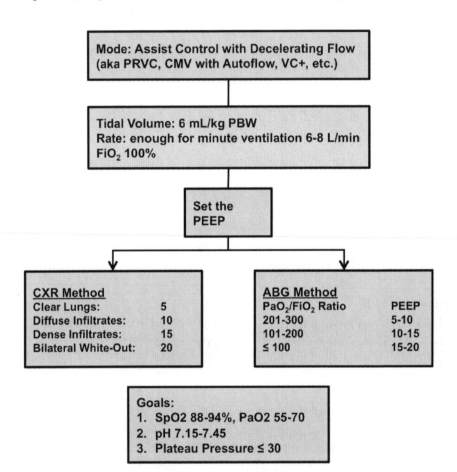

Mode: Assist Control with Decelerating Flow (aka PRVC, CMV with Autoflow, VC+, etc.)

Tidal Volume: 6 mL/kg PBW
Rate: enough for minute ventilation 6-8 L/min
FiO₂ 100%

Set the PEEP

CXR Method
Clear Lungs:	5
Diffuse Infiltrates:	10
Dense Infiltrates:	15
Bilateral White-Out:	20

ABG Method
PaO₂/FiO₂ Ratio	PEEP
201-300	5-10
101-200	10-15
≤ 100	15-20

Goals:
1. SpO2 88-94%, PaO2 55-70
2. pH 7.15-7.45
3. Plateau Pressure ≤ 30

Obstructive Lung Disease Ventilator Setup
[Status Asthmaticus, COPD, Bronchospasm]

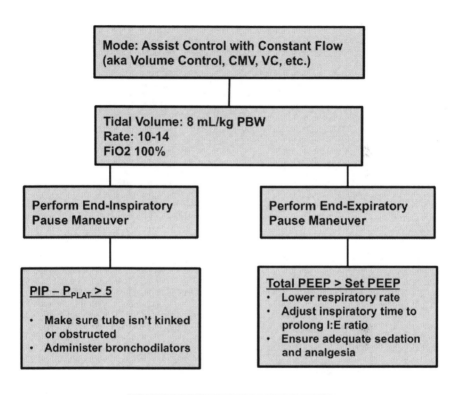

Mode: Assist Control with Constant Flow (aka Volume Control, CMV, VC, etc.)

Tidal Volume: 8 mL/kg PBW
Rate: 10-14
FiO2 100%

Perform End-Inspiratory Pause Maneuver

Perform End-Expiratory Pause Maneuver

PIP – P$_{PLAT}$ > 5

- Make sure tube isn't kinked or obstructed
- Administer bronchodilators

Total PEEP > Set PEEP
- Lower respiratory rate
- Adjust inspiratory time to prolong I:E ratio
- Ensure adequate sedation and analgesia

Goals:
1. SpO2 88-94%, PaO2 55-70
2. pH ≥ 7.10
3. I:E ratio 1:3-1:5
4. No Auto-PEEP
5. P$_{PLAT}$ ≤ 30

Consider Heliox, ketamine infusion, and therapeutic bronchoscopy if patient remains unstable

Escalating Therapy for ARDS

So here you are, at 2 A.M., and you're caring for a patient with severe ARDS. There are three things you need to know— where to start, what goals to aim for, and what to do if what you're doing isn't working.

The most evidence-based recommendation is to start with a lung-protective strategy, a la ARDSNet. Specifically, that means using lower tidal volumes (4-6 mL/kg PBW) and enough PEEP to open up and stabilize vulnerable lung units. Following the guidelines listed earlier in this chapter for acute lung injury is appropriate for initial vent settings, and adjustments should be made as necessary to achieve the listed goals. These goals include adequate oxygenation, a reasonable (but not perfect) degree of ventilation, and keeping the alveolar pressure (as represented by the plateau pressure on the vent) less than 30. If the plateau pressure exceeds 30, lowering the tidal volume to 5 or even 4 mL/kg PBW is appropriate. The respiratory rate can be increased if needed, but remember that hypercapnia is not terribly dangerous in most settings. Adjustment of the PEEP can be done using PEEP-FiO_2 tables, pressure-volume curves, esophageal pressure monitoring, or any of the other methods described in the earlier chapter.

If an ARDSNet approach isn't working, you may need to escalate. First off, however, we should define "isn't working." Most of the time, the ARDSNet ventilator management strategy is sufficient to achieve adequate oxygenation and provide lung protection. Rescue therapies like the ones discussed here do not carry strong evidence-based medicine recommendations, and should only be considered for moderate-to-severe respiratory failure. Many of the clinical trials use a PaO_2/FiO_2 ratio $\leq$ 150, which seems reasonable. For the purpose of this algorithm, "isn't working" is defined as a PaO_2/FiO_2 ratio $\leq$ 150 despite optimal treatment with the listed modality. For example, the ARDSNet approach would be considered to be "not working" if the PaO_2/FiO_2 ratio is $\leq$ 150 despite using a low tidal volume and a PEEP of 15-20. This does not mean, however, that you must try something else. A mode of ventilation or support has only failed if it can't provide the minimum necessary oxygenation for a patient, or if the adverse effects on the lungs or hemodynamics are intolerable. True refractory hypoxemic respiratory failure would be best defined as a PaO_2/FiO_2 ratio < 55 despite optimal treatment.

ARDS Escalation Algorithm

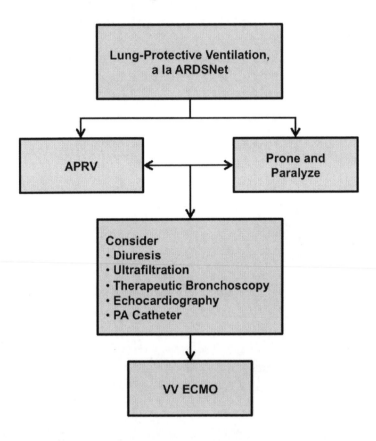

Airway Pressure Release Ventilation[*]

My go-to rescue mode of ventilation for ARDS is APRV. APRV works by increasing the mean airway pressure while avoiding excessively high distending pressure on the alveoli. It does this by going up to an inspiratory pressure (P_{HIGH}) and holding it for 3 seconds, 4 seconds, or even longer. Brief (usually less than one second) releases of airway pressure allows the gas in the patient's lungs to escape, carrying off CO_2, and the lungs are then rapidly re-expanded to the P_{HIGH}.

APRV works very well for diffuse, bilateral lung injury. It does not work as well when one lung is considerably worse than the other, and it doesn't work very well in patients with significant obstructive pulmonary disease due to the air-trapping it creates. Patients with tenuous hemodynamics may also do poorly with APRV if the distending airway pressure impacts venous return or pulmonary blood flow. APRV does seem to be well-tolerated in most patients with ARDS, however, and it has the added benefit of permitting spontaneous ventilation and not requiring heavy sedation and neuromuscular blockade.

---

[*] There's a very good chapter on APRV in *The Ventilator Book*, if I do say so myself!

APRV Setup Flowchart

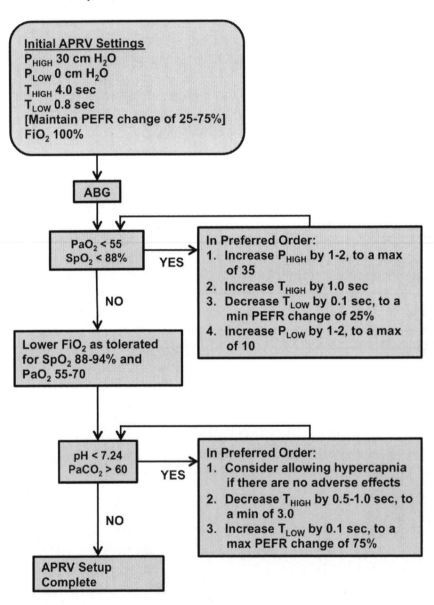

Initial APRV Settings
P_{HIGH} 30 cm H_2O
P_{LOW} 0 cm H_2O
T_{HIGH} 4.0 sec
T_{LOW} 0.8 sec
[Maintain PEFR change of 25-75%]
FiO_2 100%

ABG

PaO_2 < 55
SpO_2 < 88%

YES

In Preferred Order:
1. Increase P_{HIGH} by 1-2, to a max of 35
2. Increase T_{HIGH} by 1.0 sec
3. Decrease T_{LOW} by 0.1 sec, to a min PEFR change of 25%
4. Increase P_{LOW} by 1-2, to a max of 10

NO

Lower FiO_2 as tolerated for SpO_2 88-94% and PaO_2 55-70

pH < 7.24
$PaCO_2$ > 60

YES

In Preferred Order:
1. Consider allowing hypercapnia if there are no adverse effects
2. Decrease T_{HIGH} by 0.5-1.0 sec, to a min of 3.0
3. Increase T_{LOW} by 0.1 sec, to a max PEFR change of 75%

NO

APRV Setup Complete

Prone and Paralyze

If a patient with severe ARDS has a contraindication to APRV, or doesn't do well on APRV, I think there is sufficient evidence to recommend prone positioning (usually in conjunction with neuromuscular blockade). The success of prone positioning depends greatly on a well-trained staff and meticulous avoidance of complications like pressure injuries and dislodgement of life support devices. Therefore, using a checklist each time the patient is turned is highly recommended. Regular training of the ICU staff is also necessary. The ventilator should be kept on ARDSNet-style settings to help protect the lungs from injury, and the same goals for gas exchange apply.

If neuromuscular blockade is used, cisatracurium is the preferred agent for the reasons described in the chapter in this book. Daily interruption of the paralytic drug is advisable to avoid accumulation and prolonged neuromuscular blockade.

Patients should be prone for 16 hours, followed by 8 hours in the supine position. For both proning and paralysis, the therapy should be continued until the patient begins to show signs of recovery. Most of the time, this will mean a PaO_2/FiO_2 ratio > 150 while supine and off the paralytic agent.

Concurrent Therapy

While much of the treatment for ARDS focuses on respiratory support, it's important to recognize that volume overload, excessive pulmonary secretions, and cardiac dysfunction can also contribute to severe respiratory failure. In addition to providing optimal ventilator support, the following should be considered:

• Diuresis or ultrafiltration as tolerated, with a goal of reaching 105% of the patient's "dry weight." Volume overload is an especially common cause of persistent hypoxemia in ventilated patients.

- Therapeutic bronchoscopy to clear the tracheobronchial tree. This can also be diagnostic if the primary cause of respiratory failure is infection or alveolar hemorrhage.

- Echocardiography or a pulmonary artery catheter to identify and treat cardiac dysfunction.

Veno-Venous ECMO

VV ECMO is the ultimate rescue strategy for respiratory failure, and it works by essentially taking the lungs out of the equation so they can rest and recover. The indications for VV ECMO are outlined in the chapter in this book. VV ECMO carries very real risks—the cannulas are very large, and the anticoagulation necessary for the circuit often leads to significant bleeding and the need for multiple transfusions. It is also quite resource-intensive and can only be performed in ECMO centers. Nevertheless, VV ECMO is growing in popularity as a method of support for adults with severe respiratory failure. If a patient appears to be heading toward this and is not already at an ECMO center, early transfer should be arranged if possible.

Other Rescue Therapies

Two rescue therapies for ARDS that are not supported by the medical literature, at least in adults, are inhaled nitric oxide (iNO) and high frequency oscillatory ventilation (HFOV). That doesn't mean that they are worthless, but based on the published data, they should not be included in a general treatment algorithm.

As discussed previously in the book, iNO can be helpful for the treatment of acute right ventricular failure. For patients with ARDS, however, no mortality benefit has been described and some trials have shown an increase in harm with iNO. For that reason, the use of iNO should be limited to those patients with demonstrable acute right ventricular failure and pulmonary arterial hypertension; or, ARDS with truly refractory hypoxemia ($PaO_2/FiO_2 < 55$) when other rescue therapies have either failed or are not an option.

HFOV was, at one time, a commonly used rescue therapy. The OSCILLATE trial, published in 2013, was a multicenter trial examining the use of HFOV early in the treatment of moderate-to-severe ARDS.[37] The investigators found no evidence of benefit and a trend toward increased in-hospital mortality. This was validated by the OSCAR trial, another multicenter trial of HFOV in ARDS that found similar results.[38] For this reason, HFOV should be limited to those patients who have a specific need like a large bronchopleural fistula, or those with truly refractory hypoxemia ($PaO_2/FiO_2 < 55$) when other rescue therapies have either failed or are not an option.

HFOV Setup Flowchart

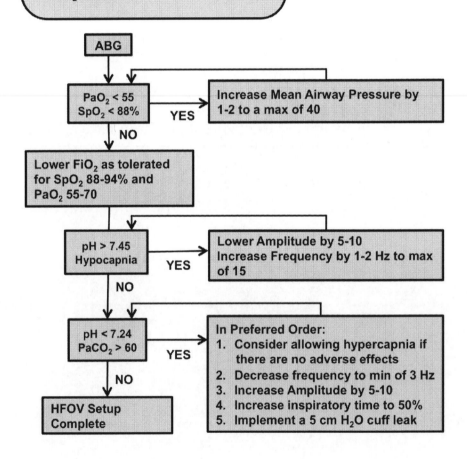

Initial HFOV Settings
- Mean Airway Pressure: 2-5 cm H_2O higher than mean airway pressure on conventional ventilation
- Amplitude: $PaCO_2$ (on last ABG) + 20
- Frequency: 5 Hz
- Inspiratory time: 33%
- FiO_2 100%

ABG

$PaO_2 < 55$
$SpO_2 < 88\%$ — **YES** → Increase Mean Airway Pressure by 1-2 to a max of 40

NO

Lower FiO_2 as tolerated for SpO_2 88-94% and PaO_2 55-70

pH > 7.45
Hypocapnia — **YES** → Lower Amplitude by 5-10
Increase Frequency by 1-2 Hz to max of 15

NO

pH < 7.24
$PaCO_2 > 60$ — **YES** → In Preferred Order:
1. Consider allowing hypercapnia if there are no adverse effects
2. Decrease frequency to min of 3 Hz
3. Increase Amplitude by 5-10
4. Increase inspiratory time to 50%
5. Implement a 5 cm H_2O cuff leak

NO

HFOV Setup Complete

References

1 Hickling KG, Henderson SJ, Jackson R. Low mortality associated with low volume pressure limited ventilation with permissive hypercapnia in severe adult respiratory distress syndrome. Intensive Care Med 16: 372–377.

2 Hickling KG, Walsh J, Henderson S, Jackson R. Low mortality rate in adult respiratory distress syndrome using low-volume, pressure-limited ventilation with permissive hypercapnia: a prospective study. Crit Care Med 22: 1568-1578.

3 Ventilation with lower tidal volumes as compared with traditional tidal volumes for acute lung injury and the acute respiratory distress syndrome. The Acute Respiratory Distress Syndrome Network. N Engl J Med 342: 1301-1308.

4 Frumin MJ, Epstein RM, Cohen G. Apneic oxygenation in man. Anesthesiology 20(6): 789-798.

5 Hotchkiss JR, Blanch L, Murias G, et al. Effects of decreased respiratory frequency on ventilator-induced lung injury. Am J Respir Crit Care Med 161: 463-468.

6 Laffey JG, O'Croinin D, McLoughlin P, Kavanagh BP. Permissive hypercapnia—role in protective lung ventilatory strategies. In Applied Physiology in Intensive Care Medicine 2 (pp. 111-120). Springer Berlin Heidelberg.

7 Akca O, Doufas AG, Morioka N, et al. Hypercapnia improves tissue oxygenation. Anesthesiology 97: 801-806.

8 Mekontso Dessap A, Charron C, Devaquet J, et al. Impact of acute hypercapnia and augmented positive end-expiratory pressure on right ventricle function in severe acute respiratory distress syndrome. Intensive Care Med 35: 1850-1858.

9 Petridis AK, Doukas A, Kienke S. et al. Acta Neurochir 152: 2143.

10 Beckman JS, Koppenol WH. Nitric oxide, superoxide, and peroxynitrite: the good, the bad, and ugly. Am J Physiol 271: C1424-C1437.

11 O'Croinin DF, Nichol AD, Hopkins N, et al. Sustained hypercapnic acidosis during pulmonary infection increases bacterial load and worsens lung injury. Crit Care Med 36: 2128-2135.

12 Higher versus lower positive end-expiratory pressures in patients with the acute respiratory distress syndrome. The National Heart, Lung, and Blood Institute ARDS Clinical Trials Network. N Engl J Med 2004; 351: 327-336.

13 Crotti S, Mascheroni D, Caironi P, et al. Recruitment and derecruitment during acute respiratory failure: a clinical study. Am J Respir Crit Care Med 2001; 164:131–140.

14 Mercat A, Richard JC, Vielle B, et al. Positive end-expiratory pressure setting in adults with acute lung injury and acute respiratory distress syndrome: a randomized controlled trial. JAMA 2008; 299:646–655.

15 Washko GR, O'Donnell CR, Loring SH. Volume-related and volume-independent effects of posture on esophageal and transpulmonary pressures in healthy subjects. J Appl Physiol 2006; 100:753–758.

16 http://www.coopersurgical.com/Products/Detail/Esophageal-Balloon-Catheter-Set

[17] Talmor D, Sarge T, Malhotra A, et al. Mechanical ventilation guided by esophageal pressure in acute lung injury. N Engl J Med 2008; 359:2095–2104.

[18] Chiumello D, Cressoni M, Carlesso E, et al. Bedside selection of positive end expiratory pressure in mild, moderate, and severe acute respiratory distress syndrome. Crit Care Med 2014; 42:252–264.

[19] Gattinoni L, Carlesso E, Brazzi L, et al. Friday night ventilation: a safety starting tool kit for mechanically ventilated patients. Minerva Anestesiol 2014; 80:1046–1057.

[20] Peters JI, Stupka JE, Singh H, et al. Status asthmaticus in the medical intensive care unit: a 30-year experience. Respir Med 2012 Mar; 106(3):344-8.

[21] Tassaux D, Jolliet P, Thouret JM, et al. Calibration of seven ICU ventilators for mechanical ventilation with helium-oxygen mixtures. Am J Respir Crit Care Med 1999;160(1): 22–32.

[22] Venkataraman, ST. Heliox during mechanical ventilation. Respir Care 2006; 51(6):632-9.

[23] Goyal S, Agrawal A. Ketamine in status asthmaticus: a review. Indian J Crit Care Med 2013; 17(3): 154-61.

[24] Strayer RJ, Nelson LS. Adverse events associated with ketamine for procedural sedation in adults. Am J Emerg Med 26(9): 985–1028.

[25] Kuyper LM, Paré PD, Hogg JC, et al. Characterization of airway plugging in fatal asthma. Am J Med 2003; 115: 6-11.

[26] Guérin C, Reignier J, Richard JC, et al, PROSEVA Study Group. Prone positioning in severe acute respiratory distress syndrome. N Engl J Med 2013; 368: 2159.

[27] Papazian L, Forel JM, Gacouin A, et al. Neuromuscular blockers in early acute respiratory distress syndrome. N Engl J Med 2010; 363: 1107-1116.

[28] Gattinoni L, Tognoni G, Pesenti A, et al, Prone-Supine Study Group. Effect of prone positioning on the survival of patients with acute respiratory failure. N Engl J Med 2001; 345: 568-573.

[29] Guérin C, Gaillard S, Lemasson S, et al. Effects of systematic prone positioning in hypoxemic acute respiratory failure: a randomized controlled trial. JAMA 2004; 292: 2379-2387.

[30] Taccone P, Pesenti A, Latini R, et al, Prone-Supine II Study Group. Prone positioning in patients with moderate and severe acute respiratory distress syndrome: a randomized controlled trial. JAMA 2009; 203: 1977-1984.

[31] Forel JM, Roch A, Marin V, et al. Neuromuscular blocking agents decrease inflammatory response in patients presenting with acute respiratory distress syndrome. Crit Care Med 2006; 34: 2749-2757.

[32] Gainnier M, Roch A, Forel JM, et al. Effect of neuromuscular blocking agents on gas exchange in patients presenting with acute respiratory distress syndrome. Crit Care Med 2004; 32: 113-119.

[33] Adhikari NK, Burns KE, Friedrich JO, et al. Effect of nitric oxide on oxygenation and mortality in acute lung injury: systematic review and meta-analysis. BMJ 2007; 334(7597): 779.

34 Adhikari NK, Dellinger RP, Lundin S, et al. Inhaled Nitric Oxide Does Not Reduce Mortality in Patients With Acute Respiratory Distress Syndrome Regardless of Severity: Systematic Review and Meta-Analysis. Crit Care Med 2014; 42: 404–12.

35 Siobal MS, Kallet RH, Pittet JF, et al. Description and evaluation of a delivery system for aerosolized prostacyclin. Respir Care 2003; 48(8): 742-753.

36 Peek GJ, Mugford M, Tiruvoipati R, et al. Efficacy and economic assessment of conventional ventilatory support versus extracorporeal membrane oxygenation for severe adult respiratory failure (CESAR): a multicentre randomised controlled trial. Lancet 2009; 374: 1351-1363.

37 Ferguson ND, Cook DJ, Guyatt GH, et al. High-frequency oscillation in early acute respiratory distress syndrome. N Engl J Med 2013; 368: 795-805.

38 Young D, Lamb SE, Shah S, et al. High-frequency oscillation for acute respiratory distress syndrome. N Engl J Med 2013; 368: 806-813.

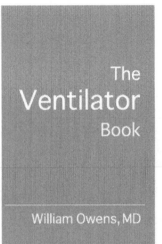

The Ventilator Book

The best-selling guide to the basics of mechanical ventilation.

Available at Amazon.com.

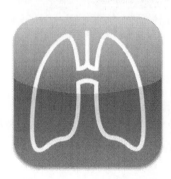

The Ventilator App

The iOS app designed to be used in the ICU or ED. It includes a tidal volume calculator, a PEEP-FiO2 adjustment tool, & a ventilator troubleshooting guide for easy reference.

Available in the App Store.

About The Author

William Owens, MD, is the Director of the Medical Intensive Care Unit at Palmetto Health Richland, a tertiary referral center in Columbia, SC. He is also the Division Chief for Pulmonary, Critical Care, and Sleep Medicine in the Palmetto Health-USC Medical Group and an Associate Professor of Clinical Medicine with the University of South Carolina. He has also served on the faculty at the University of Pittsburgh School of Medicine.

Dr. Owens is a graduate of The Citadel and the University of South Carolina School of Medicine. He trained in Emergency Medicine at the Earl K. Long Medical Center in Baton Rouge, LA. He did his fellowship training in Critical Care Medicine at the University of South Florida in Tampa, FL. He is board-certified in Emergency Medicine, Critical Care Medicine, and Neurocritical Care Medicine. He has spoken at regional and national conferences and has published articles in the peer-reviewed medical literature.

Throughout his career, Dr. Owens has been an active clinician and educator. He enjoys training physicians, nurses, and respiratory therapists in the care of the most seriously ill and injured patients and is a firm believer in a holistic approach to critical care medicine. He believes in the rational application of physiology and in always questioning our assumptions.

Dr. Owens lives in Columbia, SC, with his wife and three free-range children. He also lives with two large St. Bernards and a beehive with about 60,000 bees. He enjoys mountain biking, whitewater kayaking, playing lacrosse, and going on family adventures.

Made in the USA
Middletown, DE
06 March 2022

62214077R00073